SLAVES TO
MEDICINE

SLAVES TO MEDICINE

HOW TO RANSOM YOUR HEALTH CARE FROM
POWER & MONEY

GEORGE BEAUCHAMP, MD

Slaves to Medicine

Manufactured in the United States of America

For information, please contact:
Brown Books Publishing Group
16200 North Dallas Parkway, Suite 170
Dallas, Texas 75248
www.brownbooks.com
972-381-0009
A New Era in Publishing™

ISBN-13: 978-1-933285-94-8
ISBN-10: 1-933285-94-X
LCCN 2007935237
1 2 3 4 5 6 7 8 9 10

For Kyle, Chase, and George II—that their generation and those to follow shall not be smothered by our indulgences.

Table of Contents

Acknowledgments

This book has been a true labor of love, and I am grateful for the many people who helped make it possible by contributing their own passion for the topic.

Historically speaking, the works of Plato and Robert Pirsig have been strong influences in forming my beliefs around quality and morality in health care.

I also offer my thanks to those who have detailed the current health care disarray in more recent texts. One such contribution stands out: Maggie Mahar and her book, *Money-Driven Medicine*, provide specific context and referenced detail about how money and power have come to dominate medicine. Without her work, this book would have become unwieldy in listing the numerous recommendations for change. I consider this book a companion volume to hers.

Health economists have also pointed out the ways in which our philosophy about the economics of health care is in need of rethinking. Two deserve special comment: William Nordhaus of Yale provides the basis for the notion that health and health care are not simply costs to be endured; they are enormous contributors to a productive society. David Cutler of Harvard and his associates provide a framework for additional analysis by clarifying the economic contributions and opportunities of good health and longevity.

The Lasker Foundation analyzed the value of life and the economic consequences of improvements in both longevity and quality of life. While economics has been described as "the dismal science," there is nothing dismal about the Foundation's work. It is an amazing story of hope.

I am grateful for the privilege of caring for people as my life's work. Every day and hour, the courage and grace of the human spirit is exemplified in the practice of medicine. In an ideal world, these blessings are shared by patients, doctors, and nurses. I appreciate the many "angels" among us who lead us to healing.

Colleagues and friends tested the thoughts set forth in this book with respectful and supportive feedback. They have been more than generous with their time and invaluable insights.

Milli Brown, Kathryn Grant, the editors, and the staff of Brown Books provided the graceful refinement, shepherding, and encouragement necessary to take this manuscript from possibility to reality.

Finally, I am most grateful to my family: my parents, Kathryn and George, without whom my life likely would be misspent. My wife, Suzanne, completes my person. My daughters, Christine and Cynthia, extend their heritage, principally received from their mother, of intelligence, diligence, and courage. I have been the fortunate and undeserving recipient of their encouragement and love. This book is both a testament and a dedication to these wonderful people.

Introduction

Health care in America, by almost any standard, is in severe crisis—severe enough for one observer to call it a "death spiral." Newspaper articles speak often of the demise of the primary-care physician, describing our present health care system as too large and "dysfunctional," noting present Medicare reimbursements as roughly 30 cents on the charged dollar, and forecasting a deficit of physicians to take care of the aging population. The managed care system, with its heavy baggage of layered stakeholders, regulators, insurance companies, and agencies, has all but extinguished a primary, time-honored value of a successful health care transaction: the relationship of trust between a patient and a physician.

Unfortunately, we have reached the point where health care is in crisis, in part due to our tendency to view the relationship between patients and providers as primarily an economic relationship. Patients, however, are not merely consumers, nor are physicians solely cost centers. Physicians treat not just symptoms, but each patient as a whole person. Human medical care covers biology, social systems, and spirituality. But currently, society's interest in health care is being held hostage by power and money speculators who overrule the best interests of the many in favor of their own economic gain.

I have written this book as an urgent call to reform the present system before the forces compelling the current crisis become so threatening that only government intervention, or a forced, drastic third-party solution, can prevent collapse on a large scale. I will trace the rise of these forces that have ultimately contributed to creating the mistaken notion that health care should be treated as a cost center, with ways and means that establish a value of medical services. Most importantly, it reveals the colossal failure of this cost center model as overall expenditures for health care continue to skyrocket. What this book proposes is nothing short of a major overhaul of the entire health care system based on an entirely different set of values from the cost center model.

There is ample room to reform the health care system. With more than $2 trillion annual costs in the present system, almost $1.6 trillion may consist of spending on what are called Non-Value-Added Processes, Non-Value-Added Medicine, and self-destructive behaviors. These costs cumulate from legislators, rule-makers, bureaucrats, and enforcement agents, all the way down through insurance companies, pharmaceutical companies, and authorities in the legal system, finally ending with hospitals, doctors, and patients. These costs have been estimated as high as 80% of the total costs, and perhaps higher.

The solution I am recommending is founded upon Values-Based Medicine. It assumes that there are only two meaningful outcomes in health care: quality of life and length of life. Living well and living longer are the core outcomes in proposed health care reforms, and the new system requires measuring how well the reformed health care model envisioned performs in these two outcomes. The overall good for society can be demonstrated in economic terms by how much value extended life and a better quality of life adds to the whole economy in a measure called Economic Value Added (EVA).

If you are concerned about the future of your own personal health care, that is appropriate and rational. But you should look at the big picture, too. Our society must wake up to the fact that there is trouble brewing that threatens more than our health. Our current health care system wastes resources and fails to capitalize on the potential wealth a healthy person can create. Many people assume that a comprehensive solution will be prohibitively expensive, but investments that improve health create wealth rather than consume it. No one is exempt from a responsibility to be part of the solution to the health care dilemma. We must use our available resources to create a values-based solution that cleans up today's mess. We do not have the option to continue much further down the road we're currently walking.

This book is about creating an approach to health care that supports the three pillars of quality of life in any society: health, wealth, and liberty. They are inextricably intertwined. Change should come in the form of a values-based medicine approach—an integrated solution that springs from a belief that preserving health and providing health care is necessary for our society, our economy, and our morality.

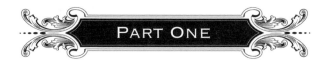

PART ONE

The Problem:
Our Medical Mess Is
Ours to Fix

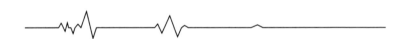

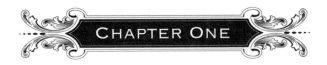

CHAPTER ONE

Health Care:
The Death Spiral

There is no wealth but life.

—John Ruskin—

The Best and Worst of Times

"It was the best of times; it was the worst of times," wrote Charles Dickens in *A Tale of Two Cities*. He could have been writing about health care today. On the bright side, medical science has never been more advanced than at present in the areas of technology, molecular genetics, pharmaceuticals, medical procedures, and medical devices. Almost daily, we read, see, and hear about breakthroughs in medicine not dreamed possible only a few years ago. We also anticipate and expect the promise of revolutionary technical improvements in patient care in the future. As a profession, medicine continues to attract persons of intellect, character, and merit. In most of these areas, the future has never looked brighter.

On the darker side, our times abound with looming problems that affect health care. Gaps in knowledge, opportunity, and wealth expand without end. Clashes between classes and cultures multiply and intensify unrelentingly. Our demands on ourselves, others, and the environment accumulate daily. Nonsense cloaked in political correctness passes for common sense. The game's the thing, and the notion of "I win, you lose" dominates the playing field. Mighty brokers of economic and political power wield influence over citizens to the point of enslavement.

All these social and economic forces gravely impact the delivery of medical care.

In modern health care, a monolithic system treats doctors, nurses, and other caregivers as interchangeable parts, as if they are all the same—a highly mechanistic view. This rigidly inflexible system, likewise, treats patients as if they are indistinguishable from one another. And the scene repels both patients and prospective caregivers alike. Dickens' words, "It was the best of times; it was the worst of times," have never seemed more true than they do today. But the dilemma of providing affordable quality health care isn't unique to our era.

Plato's "Free Men" and "Slave Doctors"

In 350 B.C.E., Plato analyzed many basic beliefs and social problems of his time, problems that reflect the same realities facing us today. Valuable clues for solving our current dilemma lie in this excerpt from The Laws, "Two Categories of Doctors," as two men discuss the predicament they face with health care:

> ATHENIAN: ". . . A state's invalids include not only free men but slaves too, who are almost always treated by other slaves who either rush about on flying visits or wait to be consulted in their surgeries. This kind of doctor never gives any account of

the particular illness of the individual slave, or is prepared to listen to one; he simply prescribes what he thinks best in the light of experience, as if he had precise knowledge, and with the self-confidence of a dictator. Then he dashes off on his way to the next slave-patient, and so takes off his master's shoulders some of the work of attending the sick. The visits of the free doctor, by contrast, are mostly concerned with treating the illnesses of free men; his method is to construct an empirical case-history by consulting the invalid and his friends; in this way he himself learns something from the sick and at the same time he gives the individual patient all the instruction he can. He gives no prescription until he has somehow gained the invalid's consent; then, coaxing him into continued cooperation, he tries to complete his restoration to health. Which of the two methods do you think makes a doctor a better healer, or a trainer more efficient? Should they use the double method to achieve a single effect, or should the method too be single—the less satisfactory approach that makes the invalid more recalcitrant?"

CLEINIAS: "The double, sir, is much better, I think."

Plato speaks of "free men" and "slave doctors." How is this any different from what exists today in regulated, managed care? When most people go to see a doctor, both the services the doctor provides and the fees that insurance companies allow him to charge are largely predetermined by parties other than the patients and doctors. Most people feel completely powerless when the time comes to submit a claim to an insurance company. They are stuck with fees negotiated by authorities higher up than they are and are not given the opportunity to have a voice in the matter. They are slaves to a master, just as people were in 350 B.C.E.

Plato also speaks of "state's invalids," who may be free men or slaves. Today's patients who receive services supported by their individual states are similar to those Plato describes. When we consider the pervasive influence of our government and the legal and regulatory control it wields over our health care, we are "state's invalids" just as people were in 350 B.C.E.

The Looming Crisis in American Health Care

Many people fail to see the looming crisis in American health care, but it is becoming harder and harder to ignore. Significant and potentially dire problems portend an unfavorable future for health care. The current debate over solutions to the crisis falls into two extremes. One side says create a highly regulated, consumer-driven health care marketplace, while the other side argues for an opposing position of a highly regulated, single-payer, government-sponsored health care system.

Both options—private or government-funded health care—contain flaws that will likely lead to failure and bear substantial risks of further erosion of our resources and liberties. Both solutions lack the most fundamental component of a successful health care system: the trust patients must have with their health care providers in order to feel that they are receiving optimal care.

Time is running out to make constructive changes in our health care system. The possibility exists that a cataclysmic event, or merely the accelerating rate of change, may soon provoke extreme measures driven by the exercise of governmental "emergency powers." More governmental intervention produces conditions likely to make matters worse. It is time for a change.

Health Care: An Accumulation of Human Relationships

The practice of medicine concerns the caring and healing relationship between a patient and a doctor. All of biology universally demonstrates the inclination of humans toward nurturing and caring, but humanity distinctively brings these traits to their highest form in a social model. Medical care is an excellent example of this social imperative. Human relationships form the only sustainable context for medical care.

Consider for a moment a wilderness devoid of any human life other than your own. In such a world, you would be completely free, and you would be completely responsible for the maintenance of your own existence. In this wilderness, there would be no health care system because there would be no one to care for you; you must provide for yourself. This observation, while patently obvious, drives home the critical point that the accumulation of many human relationships—exploring common interests, values, and caring for one another—is the foundation of health care in all its forms.

Imagine another alternative: a world comprised only of you, your doctor, and one other person, a potential intermediary. The three of you must vote on whether your health care provider will be a public servant to you, similar to a police or fire person, or an independent professional.

Which health care provider would you choose? The answer to the question determines our relationship and behavior to those who care for us in times of want or need. Clarifying the nature of this relationship, a significant task in itself, defines the type of health care system we ultimately create. If we choose to define and treat our caregivers as public servants, they become precisely that, and this choice introduces coercion. If we demand, we must command. Those we command are either preselected to servitude or conscripted to the role.

The other choice, hiring the independent professional health care provider, rests upon the presumption that human beings have many wonderful and apparently inherent characteristics. Among these characteristics, humans exhibit a significant tendency to bond with each other, subordinate their self-interests to others when appropriate, and act in virtuous ways. Hints of these characteristics are particularly demonstrated in what Mortimer Adler called the "cooperative arts": agriculture, education, and health care. This point of view supports the notion of medicine as a pursuit befitting free men and women.

The attractive option of choosing this model of an independent professional health care provider creates a choice: you can either work it out with your caregivers personally or hire a third party to do it for you. Choose the hard work of the first option and Plato would call you free; choose the ease of the second, and you will have created your version of slave medicine as Plato envisioned it.

You cannot have it both ways. You will not receive the most benefit from your relationships with your nurses and doctors if you enable insurers, regulators, administrators, and enforcers to lash them on the back. Such an encumbered system cannot long sustain benefits when it is riddled with significant waste and self-destructive behaviors. A look at current health care delivery systems, where the provision of medicine is seen as a cost center, demonstrates the consequences of third-party interference.

The Failure of Health Care as a Cost Center

In 1992, health care provision in America changed dramatically when the Resource-Based Relative Value Scale (RBRVS) became the dominant method for the determination of the marketplace value of medical services. This legislative action effectively institutionalized the "cost center" approach to health care. The trend had been moving in this direction for some time. As Congress kept adding to the beneficiaries and covered services of Medicare in the 1970s, health care, as a percentage of the federal budget, began to spin out of control. To control costs, the government undertook an analysis of the costs of providing medical services.

At the same time, within the field of medicine, additional pressures surfaced that affected costs. The American Society of Internal Medicine (ASIM) took the position that "cognitive services"—the "thinking" part of medicine, including talking to the patient, evaluating symptoms, deciding on treatment protocols—had been undervalued as compared to "procedural service" reimbursement rates. Accordingly, ASIM began a campaign to enhance the value of thinking as opposed to doing.

These two forces—cost containment and reimbursement inequities—came together to energize the creation of RBRVS. Unfortunately, the ASIM effort backfired because, in effect, the value of medical care came to be identified as the cost to provide services to recipients of Medicare. They became specified ultimately by the government. In this way, the RBRVS evolved into a system used to control and cut reimbursements for all providers. Other payers, seizing the opportunity to increase their profits, snapped into alignment with the method, and decreased reimbursements for almost all services.

Skyrocketing Health Care Expenditures

Total health care costs, however, did not go down; in fact, health care expenditures continue to skyrocket. Patients, including taxpayers and premium payers, are either paying more or dropping to uninsured and underinsured status. Provider take-home compensation continues to plummet. Profits among non-provider intermediaries are soaring, with insurance company executives' total compensation reaching hundreds of millions of dollars per year. Government regulations proliferate like rabbits. In short, the provision of health care is being ground to a halt by externally mandated, non-value-added processes (NVAPs) in the form of rules and regulations and by the waste of resources spent on non-value-adding intermediaries.

An Alzheimer's Disease Case

The following example offers insight into how we view the cost of drug treatment for Alzheimer's disease, a serious medical condition. Recently, the British health care system decertified the use of one medicine because of lack of what it deemed "proven effect." A hue and cry came forth from caregivers, who felt the drug prolonged independent living. If the person, or his family, were to pay for the medicine, or if the only consideration was demonstrated patient welfare, then the point would be moot; effective medications would be used.

The pharmaceutical industry presses insistently to have these drugs approved for use by national or managed systems of health provision. Other third-party intermediaries will have additional political, regulatory, and financial considerations, which may conflict. Political processes ascertain the voters' mood and attempt to make political capital by assuming a position of advocacy in a manner that preserves the bureaucracy. The political and regulatory mandate is limited, and promises often exceed the deliverables. The zero-sum game "preserves" resources for other purposes (and promises). Such a system inevitably distorts medical decisions directed at individual patient welfare. When these decisions are made by third parties—non-participants in clinical encounters—the best long-term investment decisions for our society will rarely be made in the interest of individual patients.

The Culprit: Medicine as a Cost Center

To gain perspective on medicine as a cost center, consider these questions and answers to a chronic health problem such as severe arthritis:

+ What would you pay to be rid of debilitating arthritis?

   Answer: You might pay a significant proportion, if not all of your net worth, if it were possible to start your life again in robust health and store up new reserves of energy, including money.

+ What do you imagine another person would be willing to invest in recovery from arthritis so that we might have a vibrant society filled with healthy people?

Answer: Society has an interest in a cure for arthritis, and it should not include a response that simply calculates how much money it can afford to throw at a problem to quiet its associated clamor.

+ If you are unable to bear the cost of recovery from arthritis, should the burden of the expense fall onto someone else?

Answer: The investment in recovery should be made by society as a whole because of the positive economic consequences of a society filled with people living healthful lives. This is especially true if a society bases this decision on its medical, human, and economic values.

+ Do you think a rational person would more readily choose to bear the full cost of recovery from arthritis if the price of treatment was clearly posted on a price list attached to the door or posted in the lobby of the doctor's office?

Answer: Some current politicians suggest that health care will be more cost-effective if prices are posted, but I think that the answer is "no."

+ Would you trust an uninformed, third party to decide which doctor you should go to for treatment of your arthritis?

Answer: I do not believe that a third party who does not know me, and who is caught between conflicts within his power-base, should be trusted with such decisions.

+ If health care is denied because of a person's age, because it is a rare disease, or by the belief of an insurance company that a particular treatment is ineffective, would you be willing to accept this denial and forego treatment?

Answer: A human life is too precious and too valuable to our economy to consider this kind of rationalization by third parties, who would be the only ones profiting from such a decision.

Who should have the authority to answer these questions? If you leave them up to third-party "health managers," you voluntarily limit your choices and freedom in exchange for "security" that only guarantees more power and money for those doing the managing, and not improvements in your health.

Our Health and Money: Inextricably Intertwined

Our social constructs condition us to what we accept as real and meaningful. In the wilderness, these constructs—health care and, particularly, wealth—have no meaning. We all have individual survival needs (basic security such as food and shelter), but our health and wealth notions exhibit their fullest meaning only in the context of a society. Health and money are inextricably intertwined and we face both great opportunity and great challenge in this realization.

Consider this simple test. Assume you have an incurable disease that will kill you tomorrow. Now, assume that a new technology can return you to perfect health for one year, but at the end of that time, you will die. What would you pay for this technology? This question has been put to many individuals. Most people would spend all they have—their entire "net worth"—for that one year of perfect health because their life is worth much more than perhaps they previously imagined.

Spending Money and Regaining Health

Most of us value our lives and health above wealth. Why, then, do we resent spending money to help maintain or regain our health?

The answer to this basic question is complex. First, we tend to adhere to the general assumption that we should be perpetually healthy. The practical side to this assumption of good health and seeing ourselves as healthy contributes to our overall well-being, which in turn actually enhances our health. Focusing on wellness, itself a natural defense mechanism, enables us to be productive and happy, rather than incessantly worrying about our inevitable demise. Wired to deny the certainty of death and the shadow of illness, our healthy denial of the potential for them ends at a perceptible boundary, a point where it becomes impossible to deny the presence of illness.

However, to presume that consistently good health is a part of the natural order of things strains logic. Considering the potential for harm from microorganisms, toxins, chemicals, mechanical hazards, floods, or fires around the globe, our expectations of living indefinitely free from harm in some way amounts to an illusion. Complete security and safety are just illusions, and if they are experienced, it is just a matter of having had a run of good luck.

A second assumption we make is that when something does go wrong with our health, it will get better by itself. Certainly, many minor illnesses and injuries heal on their own, seemingly providing evidence for this assumption. But considering the daily threats we face, we cannot sensibly expect that the body will automatically cure every possible injury by itself.

Another large part of the reason that many of us resent spending money on health care is that when we need outside intervention we think, "It's not my fault." We believe that the fault lies elsewhere and that we should not have to pay to fix the problem. Society cultivates "not my fault" thinking, but this concept is naïve. To some degree sustained health and welfare are granted, but after that, they are earned. We must acknowledge our own roles in producing poor health and injury from smoking, overeating, under-exercising, careless driving, and other unsafe habits. There are costs to all our behaviors.

We must also acknowledge that even when we are not at fault—when we are suffering from disease or injury that we have had no part in producing—we are still responsible for regaining and maintaining good health. If we assume that all the problems we experience are someone else's to fix, we forfeit the right to contribute to the solution. In fact, we wield considerable power in maintaining and restoring our own good health. When we give up our personal responsibility and relegate it to someone else, we squander the power of this freedom. No one has a greater stake in our health than we do.

Other reasons for the reluctance to include health care expense in our individual budgets include such ideas as, "I deserve the care" (i.e., "I have a legitimate need or disability") or "I've already paid for it by my labor at work, which is worth more than I'm paid," or "I've paid for it by my taxes, my good deeds, or by surviving to my current age."

Compare this mentality with our view of paying for other things that we need. Even though we have worked hard, we do not expect to receive appliances for which we have not paid. Our taxes do not pay for television repairs. Our material desires are not guaranteed because of kindness, age, or disability. We do not expect to avoid paying for repairing or replacing old cars, out-of-style clothes, or other belongings. Natural wear and tear occurs on all things, and few, if any, are replaced at no cost to us. Is it rational that what we value most—our health—is what we seem most reluctant to spend our own money on?

Cost Center Mentality: The Nexus of the Problem

Imagine the managed care approach to the health care system applied to other aspects of society. What if we had a "managed" food service? A person would go to the grocery store and select—or claim to need—$250 worth of food. At checkout, the customer would offer $30 as a "co-payment" and then instruct the grocer to collect their "allowed" charges from a third party.

Let us say that the allowed charges are $150. Now, the grocer must charge its cash customers $400 to cover the loss incurred by the "managed" customer, plus all the non-value-added processes of creating, filling out, and processing forms, postage, and the value of discounted and delayed payments. Does this sound like a viable system? Why would we expect a similar system for health care to run smoothly? Government-subsidized and government-enabled attempts to control the health care system through the so-called private markets provide the nexus of the problem.

When we relegate the financial responsibility for our health to someone else, we automatically discount health care expenditures to the status of a "cost center." Considering medicine as a cost center for which others should pay, and not an investment in the well-being of one's own society, is a fundamental flaw in the American health care system. It is simply too easy to spend someone else's money. The distinction between needs and wants blurs. We lose sight of what is vital versus what is excessive. Political ideas are forged from an artificial and false premise to demand and enforce protocols that unnecessarily drain resources. To compensate for the strain, the system must undergo relentless cost cutting. When cost cutting reigns, quality is chipped, eroded, and squeezed until the final product bears slim resemblance to its ideal. The ultimate result of the cost center mentality is inferior quality in preserving or restoring that which is most precious to us as individuals—our health. Holman W. Jenkins, Jr., summarizes the necessary sequence of reform in health care. We must move "toward greater reliance on individual responsibility than on the illusory freelunchism of government transfers. For the problem of Medicare is the problem of health care writ small: The illusion that somebody else is available to pay our bills for us" (A14).

Government payers and insurers, the purveyors of this cost-cutting mentality and strategy, also have structural conflicts of interest. Any money "saved" through cuts is an opportunity either to apply those monies to fulfill additional political promises or to add to their profitability.

We must understand this reality: cutting costs ultimately means cutting health care and limiting economic growth. In the end, the cost-cutting mentality is counter-intuitive to rational human nature and just plain self-destructive. Health is extremely valuable, and our doctors and nurses help deliver that value. It is ironic that the provider community is most often blamed for rising costs in health care. Government and insurers nod at quality of care and then treat it as a tool for discipline, a means for restriction of reimbursement, or an excuse for greater regulation.

This is the inevitable result of a model that rewards doctors and nurses on the basis of doing things, dispensing things, or spending time, rather than creating value. It is also the result of a regulatory and payer mindset, which assumes that some things must be excessive and those things must be cut.

Two derivative forces are at work today. One is "Pay for Performance." According to Congress, doctors need to demonstrate that they are providing high quality care for the money they "take." The best measure of the quality of a medical treatment is, of course, its outcome. However, ways of measuring outcomes are not clearly understood or well-developed, and thus measurements of processes are generally substituted. The government and payers decide which processes need to be measured and what will be considered adequate performance. We should acknowledge that, in gaining consensus on quality measures, the results are generally "lowest-common-denominator" process measures and have been one of the bases for "an arcane payment system that for decades has held back efforts to improve care" (Rosenthal 2007, 743). Providers are burdened with demonstrating adherence to these mandated processes, which may have no meaning in regard to what outcomes are actually achieved. Providers are then punished with additional overhead expenses to justify their existence by way of processes that are at best indifferent to outcomes of care. Persisting in the current strategy that provider compensation should be continually "cut," and the societal value of their compensation shredded, means consequences that are not healthy to individuals or to the vitality of society. Is society benefited more by an actor paid $1 million per episode to play a brain surgeon on TV than the value of a real brain surgeon?

The second federal congressional mechanism in place today is the "Sustainable Growth Rate" (SGR), a budget management strategy to prolong, but not assure, the future of Medicare through limiting reimbursements to providers in accordance with a formula that links projected budget revenues to payments. Note the absence of reference to quality or any other moral or ethical value. This is merely a calculation of what revenue is expected over a period of time. For example, over the next six years, the SGR is projected to cut reimbursements to physicians by an average of 39%. This is not likely to make the average beneficiary feel comfortable about the future availability of physicians to care for them. Untold resources will be wasted in the yearly "dance" as physicians and their representatives seek a "fix" to the SGR, only to return the following year in increasingly strident refrains. The system's combination of Pay for Performance and SGR has both patients and providers on the rack.

Both corporate and government actions, beliefs, and attitudes have produced the present monolithic cost-dominated system for the provision of medical services, a firmly entrenched system that will not be reformed easily. In a public exchange, one of Jan Carlzon's business school professors refreshed the lesson: "We only taught you one thing at business school—reduction of costs" (Peters 1985, 63). Such a model leaves the health care system positioned for only one type of business strategy—cost cutting—either by cutting reimbursements or by cutting provision of services. The end result can only be some combination of rationing of services or "forced labor" of servant providers with eventual cataclysmic systemic failure. The next chapter examines in depth the results gleaned from "following the money" in health care and further demonstrates the need for widespread, systemic reform.

References

Jenkins, Holman W. 2007, February 7. "The Biggest Secret in Health Care." *Wall Street Journal*. A14.

Peters, Tom and Nancy Austin, 1985. *A Passion for Excellence*. New York: Random House.

Plato, 1970. *The Laws*. "Two Categories of Doctors." New York: Penguin Classics.

Rosenthal, Meredith B. and R. Adams. 2007, February 21. "Pay-for-Performance: Will the Latest Payment Trend Improve Care?" *JAMA* 297, No 7:740-743.

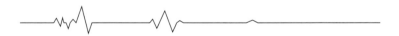

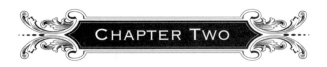

CHAPTER TWO

The American Health Care Crisis: Follow the Money

The life and liberty and property and happiness
of the common man throughout the world are at
the absolute mercy of a few persons whom he has
never seen, involved in complicated quarrels that
he has never heard of.

—Gilbert Murray—

The League of Nations and the Democratic Idea

The Dysfunctions of "Money-Driven" Medicine

Money functions poorly as either the driver or the end point in health care. In *Money-Driven Medicine*, Maggie Mahar comprehensively summarizes the forces driving medicine today; its dynamics, counter-dynamics, texts, and subtexts (Mahar 2006, 27). At their lowest common denominator, these forces all boil down to one major element: money.

Money drives health care away from the traditional relationships of values and trust, and this powerful economic force transforms the whole system into a business and industry model. The business model of industrial and market forces—particularly supply and demand—do not work well in health care, which is a "cooperative art," not a traditional "industry." Treating health care as a commodity that responds to market influences does not make sense for several reasons.

Health care cannot accurately be defined as a service in the usual economic sense of the word because market forces tend to drive demand inappropriately. A market-driven health care system leads to the overuse of technology and procedures for some health care recipients and the systematic under use for others, generally the poor and uninsured. Perverse incentives lead to perverted practices. The deeper truth is that "what is good for business is more business," but more business is not necessarily good for health care (Mahar 2006, 27).

The ultra-competitive health care marketplace subverts the fundamental cooperative and collaborative values of medicine, a competition leading to waste and inefficiency. Moreover, the system diverts enormous sums of money to those who divide value rather than create it. This competition produces an environment rife with short term concerns—an improvident approach in a field requiring a long-term commitment. In an environment of constant consolidation, acquisition, and divesture, powerful economic forces produce destabilizing change in this marketplace. At the same time, patient interests get lost in stirring the pot for profit and using the shine of the deal to trump up shareholder value. Along the way, the hyping of supply creates waste through marketing of unproven procedures. The same hype drives revenue through volume and makes waste of what suppliers have created.

The dysfunctions of money-driven medicine provoke widespread concerns about the quality of American health care, principally voiced by physicians and nurses, who have been pushed to the outer limits of health care. We do too much for some patients, but not enough for others. Marketing and supply distribution differences

between geographical areas drives a widening gap
between what are necessary and sufficient value-added
health care services. In the alternative, individual medical necessity and best medical practices, delivered in
a social context of trust, are much more likely to be
humanly and economically beneficial.

A culture filled with political and ethical dilemmas permeates our health care system, raising significant questions:
Is health care a right or a privilege? Does quality of care
equate to equality of outcome? Other perplexing dilemmas include whether care should be rationed, whether
we face a scarcity of health care resources, and whether
prices should be controlled or market-driven.

The central truth repeatedly overlooked in discussion
of these issues concerns the nature of health care itself.
Health care is a relationship based on trust. Without
trust, the nature of the profession and its valued outcomes are inevitably perverted. Trust erodes when market forces, political control, and enforced, third-party
interests collide in health care. To regain trust, physicians
and nurses must once again be placed in positions of
authority, creating a morality—quality of care—based on
competence. That trust may be sustained only when the
caring professional subordinates his or her interests to
those of the patient. These patient interests should not

be served primarily by third parties, who use power and money to increase their ultimate control. As a massive shift in power to corporations has progressed—driven by short-term profit and shareholder returns—patient care has been enslaved to profiteering.

The Flood of Rising Costs and Reduced Benefits

Despite dramatic and dangerous cuts in reimbursement to health care providers by private and government health care payers, health insurance premiums and government health care costs continue to rise rapidly at unsustainable rates. American manufacturers complain that the health costs of their employees and retirees constitute a major factor in their loss of competitiveness with the rest of the world. Americans continue to drop health insurance due to high premiums and poor coverage.

Increasingly patients, frustrated at the rising costs and reduced benefits, blame their physicians for the high costs. They believe they are receiving lower quality care despite paying higher insurance premiums. Physicians must see more patients in less time, leading to patient frustration and deteriorating patient-physician relation-ships. Managed care erodes patient loyalty through group dealing and restricting choices. These factors contribute to the worsening malpractice crisis and feed the increases in malpractice premiums.

On January 30, 2006, The American College of Physicians warned, "Primary care is on the verge of collapse. Few young physicians are going into primary care, and those already in practice are under such stress that they are looking for an exit strategy." Unfortunately, their proposed solution involved more controls, more bureaucracy, and less access to specialists.

A common perception persists that technology has increased the costs of health care and that new ways must be developed to control costs. This mistaken perception pervaded some of the premises behind managed care, Resource-Based Relative Value Scales (RBRVS), and other complex systems designed to control health care. The facts do not support this conclusion. For many diseases, technology remarkably reduced the cost of care and improved both the quality of care and the quality of patient life. This misinterpretation of technology in medicine represents a common flaw in the logic applied to health care: a false premise leading to flawed conclusions and misdirected action.

Both patients and care providers look to government for a solution, but the current $2 trillion-plus annual U.S.

health care expenditure seems already too great to manage. Medicaid, Tricare, and Medicare reimbursements often fall below the standard necessary to sustain quality health care. Government plans additional cuts scheduled to take effect over the next five years. Federal deficits likewise threaten the general welfare, apparently permitting no room to increase the budget for health care. Although the present conditions described sound grim, the future looks even worse.

The Money Path: Patient Care Shorted

Let us take a look at how health care spending is distributed. Where is the money going? Good forensic accounting suggests that to find the infractions and flaws, "follow the money." In health care, the picture is muddled because economic data is very hard to acquire. But one thing emerges clearly from what is known: most of the money paid out is not spent on patient care. Most of it goes to support the system and its intermediary power and money brokers.

Maggie Mahar systematically surveys the costs of health care by sector (Mahar x,xi). By looking at the two charts which follow, we see clearly who pays for health care in America and what health care functions receive the lion's share of the total.

WHAT WE ARE PAYING FOR

+ Private insurers' profits and administrative costs 4.5%

+ Administrative costs of government programs 2.2%

+ Nursing home care 7%

+ Prescription drugs (sold directly to patients) 11%

+ Physicians and other clinical services 22%

+ Miscellaneous dental, home health, over-the-counter medicines 22%

+ Hospital care 31%

WHO IS PAYING

+ TAXPAYERS: Medicare 17%

+ TAXPAYERS: Medicaid and SCHIP 18%

+ TAXPAYERS: Veterans' programs, public hospitals, schools 12%

+ TAXPAYERS: Private insurance for government employees 8%

+ PRIVATE INSURANCE: Employer-employee and self-employed 30%

+ PATIENTS: Out-of-pocket 14%

+ CHARITY and PHILANTHROPY: (including capital construction) 5%

FIG. 2.1 SOURCE: MAHAR, MAGGIE. 2006.
MONEY-DRIVEN MEDICINE.

The health care industry and the bureaucracy accept Mahar's distribution of resources, yet the numbers do not tell the whole story. These numbers fail to clarify and disclose all the money spent on the provider side of the system. While 22% goes to physicians and 31% to hospitals, the proportion of these numbers diverted to Non-Value-Added Processes (NVAPs) prior to, or instead of, patient care lies obscured and difficult to uncover. The actual amounts of these costs actually paid to persons taking care of patients remain unknown. In fact, these NVAP expenditures likely become obscured or entirely hidden in creative accounting. If, for example, physicians actually received 22% of the $2 trillion health care pie, then every licensed physician in the country, including those not in clinical practices, would be paid an average annual income of $650,000. In reality, the average physician's income fails to reach this number by fractions less than half.

Physicians actually keep only one quarter to one third of the monies paid to them. Most of the rest goes to paying for, and dancing to, payer and regulatory tunes. In the hospital sector of health care, where power, regulatory structures, and requirements consume inordinate resources, finding the data becomes even more difficult to pinpoint. Perhaps as much as two of every three dollars spent caring for patients goes to these NVAP expenditures.

Superimpose the wrong-headed notions and requirements of "fostering competition," or more accurately, "festering competition," and the provider system emerges as alarmingly dysfunctional in its wastefulness.

The remaining sectors of the industry experience their own dysfunction. Dr. Irene Ludwig's surveys of the health care system probe two critical questions of cost. First, what percent of health care system costs, covered by insurance premiums or tax dollars, constitutes the expenses for overhead or bureaucracy? Second, what percentage of these covered amounts actually goes to direct patient care? According to Dr. Ludwig's survey, providers in academia or hospital-based practices without direct contact with a business office estimate overhead at 50-60%; private practitioners estimate 50-90%; younger practitioners, nurses, and ancillary personnel estimate 80-90%, the highest of all (Ludwig 2006). Health policy experts generally estimate significantly lower percentages.

The health advisor to the Governor of New York, medical economists in congressional offices, hospital CEOs, and others, generally place the figure at 25-30%. A leading legal firm that advises hospitals on health policies puts the number at 40% (Ludwig 2006). A substantially wider gap exists between the estimates supplied by active health providers and policy decision-makers. What accounts for the lower numbers of the policy experts may be self-serving, optimistic, and overly enthusiastic interests, rather than the reality of the costs.

The truth is that nobody knows how many dollars entering the health care system actually go to overhead, bureaucracy, or patient care. Those making the policy decisions affecting all of us continue grossly to underestimate the costs of bureaucracy, based on flawed economic assumptions and perhaps their own industry view. For example, a hospital classifies a nurse as a care provider. But an operating room circulating nurse spends on average 90% of his or her time at the computer feeding data into the information and financial systems and should be classified as 90% bureaucrat. Most physicians spend at least 40% of their time on non-direct patient care activities, including dictating, charting, insurance issues, credentialing, and mandated training and should be considered as 40% bureaucrat. Hospitals do not break down the time of their employees in this fashion. Detailed time studies would be required to get this information and it will likely remain obscured without significant external influence or investment.

The cost of medical equipment exerts considerable impact on patient care costs. A manufacturer of electrophysiological equipment attributes 50% of the cost of each device directly to unnecessary bureaucratic requirements. He sells the exact same equipment for animal research at half the price.

Patient care costs of prescription drugs by no means escape these bureaucratic and overhead add-on costs. You may be surprised to learn that clinical trials and studies do not comprise the majority of the costs for the research and development (R&D) of prescription drugs. The majority of cost comes in paperwork needed to gain Federal Drug Administration (FDA) approval. Considering that marketing exceeds all of R&D by a factor of three to four combined with the potential for litigation, you can see that bureaucracy drives most of the costs. The same dynamic applies to implantable devices.

Health care system providers themselves add to the sources of bureaucratic and regulatory costs through vast professional networks and affiliations. Providers contribute to overhead through self-generated recertification, specialty boards, institutional review boards, hospital committees, defensive medicine, professional organizations, compliance with the Resource-Based Relative Value System (RBRVS), International Classification of Disease codes (ICD, World Health Organization), Current Procedural Terminology (CPT, American Medical Association), documentation to maintain malpractice insurance, preferred practice guidelines and compliance, quality assurance committees, inter-specialty conflicts, and now Pay for Performance or euphemistically, Value-Based Purchasing for Medicare Services. The list appears endless and continues to expand.

Government-imposed rules and regulations comprise a veritable alphabet soup of regulation, including the Emergency Medical Treatment and Active Labor Act (EMTALA), Health Insurance Portability and Accountability Act (HIPAA), Stark (I, II, III; Federal Anti-Kickback Statutes), Federal Drug Administration (FDA), Centers for Disease Control (CDC), Diagnosis Related Groups (DRG) coding and reimbursement, medical licensure, continuing medical education (CME), complex requirements for exam coding levels, and most recently, the Medicare Modernization Act (MMA). If you want to know more about these regulations, please consult the medical librarian at your local hospital; he or she will guide you to a world in which you will quickly become both disoriented and repulsed by the complexity of the waste.

If a provider alters optimum patient care, such as performing an unnecessary test to satisfy a guideline rather than in order to facilitate diagnosis, that test constitutes both a bureaucratic exercise and an unnecessary cost. The system harms the patient, creates waste, misuses resources, and erodes trust.

Industry also imposes significant bureaucratic burdens on providers, including managed care, billing costs, credentialing, and malpractice defense. Health insurers add large costs to the system, probably eating up to 30% or more of each health care dollar. Independent regulatory agencies with their own alphabet soup— Joint Commission for the Accreditation of Health Related Organizations (JCAHO), National Center for Quality Assurance (NCQA), Healthstream (CME), and Graduate Medical Education (GME) committees—all pursue compliance with a set of rules that are often difficult to connect to actual patient care outcomes, and which first provide for the perpetuation of their own existence. Hospitals and medical schools also sustain large bureaucracies.

State laws govern the peer review and scope of privilege matters. Other bureaucracies affecting all businesses impose governmental burdens of varying costs in the highly labor-intensive health care field. These include the Occupational Safety and Health Administration (OSHA), tax laws, anti-discrimination policies, and a vast array of contract law. The new Medicare drug plan (MMA) subsidizes companies in creating new complexity with the lure of large profits, which increases share prices and shareholder returns while adding no value.

In short, the "industry" spawns new cost centers with each new regulatory initiative, including consultants, software companies, and additional insurance products, while patient care contracts. While no one disagrees with meaningful performance measurement, more regulation leads to more cost. Providers become frustrated and patients lose trust. Neglect of patient care and patient interests mount as money wasted on matters of tangential relevance to patient care breeds contempt for the entire health care system, creating a merry-go-round that no one can stop.

Big, Wasteful, Inefficient Business

Whether or not we define health care as an "industry," it has become big business. Large hospital management corporations show record profits. They tout lower costs by improving efficiency but also skim large sums from the system. Thousands of health-related companies and corporations generate impressive earnings, again with few credible claims for patient care value. Health insurers, companies managing CME, billing and auditing, consultants, medical marketing, public relations, lawyers, Independent Practice Associations (IPAs), billing and credentialing companies, and accounting firms—all thrive in the government-subsidized adversarial pot.

We pay a significant cost for all this bureaucracy. Dr. Ludwig estimates the percentage of non-patient, health care-related expenditures to be 85% of the total; I conservatively estimate the percentage of waste at 60%, meaning NVAP costs—people and processes not directly beneficial to patient outcomes. I divide this waste into three categories of expenses, each comprising approximately one third of the total.

+ The first 20% is spent by medical providers on administration of the facilities, personnel, keeping in compliance with payer requirements, billing and collecting, as well as the costs of internal staffing to review contracts and track payer behavior. This 20% may be a serious underestimate of the true costs of these NVAPs.

+ The second 20% reflects those costs that we pay to the system for the administration and profit of non-patient-care-related entities, including health bureaucracies, political processes, payer processes, and their profit. This 20% may also be a gross underestimate of the true costs. There is a long list of bureaucratic exercises and expenses imposed on medical practice. The only industry in America that is more regulated than health care is nuclear power. Most insurance companies report their "medical loss ratio"—the money actually reimbursed to care providers that care for patients—as a key performance indicator. The lower the ratio, the more money and profit stays with the insurance company. Numbers under 80% are considered standard, but they prefer that the number be closer to the mid-70th percentile.

+ The third 20% spent on NVAPs includes the costs of legal protection, the cost of what payors and enforcers call "fraud and abuse," and the costs imposed on providers for regulatory compliance with Medicare, OSHA, Stark, EMTALA, HIPAA, and state laws.

This means that we will have spent about $1.2 trillion (60% of $2 trillion) this year and no patient has yet received any care!

This waste is indefensible, both as a business investment and on moral grounds. That number rises substantially when waste is further defined as expenses incurred to treat self-inflicted diseases, which are theoretically avoidable. Estimates suggest that a minimum of half of monies expended in the care of disease are spent on self-inflicted disease. This category includes persons who smoke, neglect weight control, fail to exercise, ignore seatbelts, and refuse to take effective medicines.

In addition to the costs of excessive and unnecessary procedures, unproven and ineffective procedures also exert tremendous cost pressures on the system. Jack

Wennberg, M.D., estimates that these procedures consume one-third of health care dollars (Mahar 2006, 159). Collectively, these ineffective and unproven procedures may be called Non-Value-Added Medicine (NVAM). Don Berwick, M.D., estimates that, "The waste level in health care approaches 50%" (Galvin). The uneven distribution of health care spending represents another problem. A relatively small percentage, 30% of Americans, account for 90% of all the spending. This spending originates primarily from Medicare, chronic disease, and geographic variations including certain high intensity markets.

Although figures do not lie, they certainly can be used to support a variety of perspectives. By simply following the money, yet another application of the "80-20 rule" emerges. We can conclude that approximately 20% or less of the money does the work of caring for irreducible disease and that the remaining 80% or more of the money constitutes waste from NVAPs, NVAM, and bad behavior. I explore this topic further in chapter 3.

Risks and Rewards

When we follow the money, the notion of risk, whether economic or medical, raises several questions. Who is at risk? Does health insurance diminish risk, and if so, of what type? The answer to the first question is that the only real risk to a person's health is within that person, and collectively, the risk is to society. The answer to the second and third questions is that it is common practice for third parties to market their ability to assume risk on behalf of a so-called "beneficiary." An insurance company ostensibly assumes a financial risk to insure a beneficiary's health. Each of these premises should be carefully examined and called into question. Insurance companies currently take essentially no financial risk. They function with highly sophisticated business strategies and actuarial tools to offer their policies as products that primarily guarantee that they will be profitable, like bookmakers. If they are not sufficiently profitable, premiums are increased or reimbursements are decreased until they are profitable. They assume no medical risk because they contractually engineer it out of their system. Where's the benefit?

Government superficially appears to take some financial risk as a substantial payer for health services; however, taxpayers ultimately pay these bills, and debt and taxes rise to cover the expenses. Governments and bureaucracies first and foremost take care of and perpetuate themselves and their power.

Big corporations do not pay taxes, despite a fantasy to the contrary. Businesses and corporations collect taxes from employees and customers. They have vulnerabilities, but they are largely political, hence the large amounts of money they spend to curry special-interest favors.

If the government should default on its health care obligations, there would be no recourse for citizens. There is no real financial risk for government; the risks of health and its economic burdens ultimately are our risks. There is no protection against disease other than that which we provide for ourselves, or those provided by our environment and our caregivers. When we buy insurance coverage we limit our financial exposure by pre-paying at a premium, or perhaps (we may even hope), transferring the financial obligation to someone else. The economical and social costs are very high for this delusion of safety. We cannot transfer our medical risk because it is ours to bear.

As part of a legacy of employer-sponsored health care, some assume they, particularly corporations, should bear some of the financial risk for their employees' health. Some do, and even provide on-campus health care services. Other corporations take the position that this is simply a cost of doing business, and one that is mitigated by the taxes they pay.

In any discussion of risk, there are inevitably questions about reward, such as whom, what, and how much should be rewarded for bearing the risk? How much of it should go to those whose productivity must sustain the investments required to achieve and maintain good health, namely citizens themselves? How much should go to those inside the health care system who are actually taking care of patients? How much of it should go to those who control both of these groups? How about cultural and political models such as victimhood and rights? These and other related questions will need to be answered.

The Urgent Need for Reform

Michael Porter and Elizabeth Olmsted Teisberg, authors of *Redefining Health Care*, recently added a new perspective on health care, highlighting the need for health care reform. "The US health system," they say, "has the wrong kind of competition. We have a zero-sum competition to assemble bargaining power, shift the cost to others, grab more of the revenue versus other actors in the system, and restrict services. . . ." Almost everybody continues to lose in this competitive system.

Porter and Teisberg offer an entirely different approach to competition in health care:

> "Competing on value must revolve around results. The results that matter are patient outcomes per unit of cost at the medical condition level. Competition on results means that those providers, health plans, and suppliers that achieve excellence are rewarded with more business, while those that fail to demonstrate good results decline or cease to provide that service. Competition to shift cost and limit services is a zero-sum competition—one actor's gain is a loss for others. Competing on patient results is a positive-sum competition from which all system participants benefit. When providers succeed in delivering superior value, patients win, employers win, and health plans also win through better outcomes achieved at lower costs. . . . The best way to achieve lower costs is actually to drive up quality. That's the dynamic we need to harness. [And then] the US system can be reformed from the bottom up." (Porter and Teisberg 2006, 37-38)

Although Porter and Teisberg accurately characterize much of the dysfunction in the current health care system, their solution and line of argument present certain problems that will be difficult, if not impossible, to resolve. First, meaningful quality must be achieved in medicine at the level of the whole person (patient) and not at some intermediate "medical condition" level. Second, the notion of "competition for quality" causes problems that may more likely render it an empty turn of phrase rather than a sustainable strategy.

Real quality improvements require collaboration, not competition. The interests of patients and caregivers can only be meaningfully aligned through cooperative efforts. Competition in this context not only implies, but requires, a third party to state the rules of engagement, referee, keep score, set rewards, and compel the participants to conform to the third-party's interests. Non-zero-sum outcomes are characteristic of cooperative efforts, not competitive ones. Their rhetoric is revealing when they say that "driv(ing) up quality (is) the dynamic we need to harness."

Their imagery of driving and harnessing conjures up the notion of Plato's slave medicine with its consequences. This imagery sounds and appears explicitly contradictory: compel the parties to compete; harness them to the task! It will not work, and we will be further enslaved by the effort. Finally, the hopeful assertion that the system may be "reformed from the bottom up" by competing for value seems inconsistent with the reality of who would drive the process just described. You cannot drive reform from the bottom up if the bottom must serve master interests.

The authors' stated belief that room exists for all current stakeholders, including health plans, in their new compete-for-quality marketplace sounds unrealistic and even Pollyannaish. Even they acknowledge that "Health plans have eroded the trust of many subscribers during the era of gate-keeping, denial of claims, and restricted networks." What an understatement!

To say that health plans have also "eroded the trust" of doctors and nurses would be another colossal understatement. Nonetheless, the authors continue to suggest that "because health plans have important value-adding roles in the system, such as collecting results information, advising patients, and referring physicians," they should have an ongoing role, including being "the logical place in the system at which to aggregate medical records."

Let us see, then, that (other than their employees and shareholders) health plans have "eroded" nearly everyone's trust! Why should we trust them to "add value" by advising doctors and patients and being the keeper of our collective records? Where is the basis for that conclusion?!

The urgent need to reform this system weighs more heavily upon us than ever. The health care system currently positions hospitals, physicians, nurses, and other secondary medical professional groups tragically and wastefully to squabble over an ever-shrinking slice of the so-called health care pie, a pie defined by third-party interests. At best, it is an unintended consequence. But it is more likely that those prospering from the current system conspire to create this reality. Meanwhile, controlling entities consume the bulk of the pie, while the overall problem worsens. We should no longer stand for this.

As we look to potential health care solutions, the waste in the current system will require an overhaul. The longer we try to cope within this corrupt system, the worse the collapse will be and the more prolonged the recovery. The situation, however, is definitely not hopeless. We can rearrange our priorities, or more accurately, we can rearrange our behavior, in a way that is more in alignment with what our philosophical and cultural priorities already are. Since we value our lives and health above other assets, we can begin to view medicine as a value production center rather than a cost center.

There is compelling evidence that good health, including that derived from good health care, is highly contributory to individual lives, communities, and economies. These valued contributions include improved quality of life, increased longevity, and the consequential increased productiveness that accompanies economic growth and vitality. To the degree that this is so, we are likely to be seriously under-investing in health and health care, a wasteful behavior. The benefits of relatively modest investments in effective health care services are highly leveraged, and the results far exceed any other investment we can make. This reality of life is being subverted by short-term, power-based, and money-based forces. Chapter three looks at the distribution of power and responsibility in the provision of health care and how giving away power affects the quality of care provided.

References

Galvin, Robert. 2005, January 12. A Deficiency of Will and Ambition? A Conversation with Donald Berwick. Web Exclusive. *Health Affairs.*

Ludwig, Irene. Personal Communication.

Mahar, Maggie. 2006. *Money-Driven Medicine.* New York: Harper Collins Publishers.

Porter, Michael and Elizabeth Olmsted Teisberg. 2006. *Redefining Health Care.* Boston: Harvard University Press.

Porter, Michael and Elizabeth Olmsted Teisberg. 2006, September. *HBS Alumni Review* (an interview), 37-38.

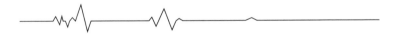

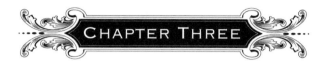

CHAPTER THREE

Power and Responsibility: Yours, Ours, Theirs

One of America's most cherished political illusions is that we all receive the same health care regardless of income. The reality is very different. A change is needed and we have the power to bring it about.

—Dr. John Kitzhaber—

Former Governor of Oregon

Politics and Power-Driven Medicine

Notions of entitlement currently dominate our culture and our politics. We justify entitlement on the basis of "rights" and codify it in both law and social correctness. In turn, "rights" unfortunately can be perverted as a rationale for tapping the property of others and for creating mechanisms to coerce others to share their resources. A self-perpetuating whirlpool of power, law, regulation, bureaucracy, and enforcement feeds off the liberties of those people who claim entitlement from the resources and liberty of taxpayers and providers. The consequence of this powerful cycle creates what Fareed Zakaria in *The Future of Freedom* calls "illiberal democracy." Zakaria describes a worldwide trend of democracies becoming the opposite of liberal (free) and, instead, infringing on the liberties of citizens through so-called democratic methods of power enforcement. In a perverted, ironic sense, a superficial and unsustainable social tranquility is purchased and imposed by the process at the sacrifice of liberty.

This whirlwind of power engulfs medicine. Culture drives politics, politics drives the economic system, and the imperatives of the political system drive medical practice and delivery. This cycle leaves medicine in a highly dependent position, driven by forces which do not necessarily assign fair or reasonable values to the practice, nor protect the medical or human interests of patients.

Democratically Imposed, Slow-Motion Tyranny

The current power model can be demonstrated by a scenario involving three people. Consider party A, who claims a "right" that requires the resources of another party for its fulfillment, party B. Party B has the resources and may be willing to share them up to a point for the preservation of a tranquil society. When party B shares, he shares from a highly principled standpoint, fulfilling the Golden Rule, classical virtues, and charity.

When A's demands exceed B's resources and willingness to voluntarily share them, A's call on B's resources creates strain and becomes unworkable. Then party A either physically removes the resources by stealing them away or calls upon party C to force party B to share resources by so-called lawful capture, a type of eminent domain. In the theft scenario, the result is violent tyranny. In the political enforcement scenario, a transaction results whereby A trades something of value to C, usually a vote, a tax payment, or a premium.

All these values represent pieces of A's liberty. In return for the acquisition of this power at the price of A's liberties, party C makes a call on party B to comply with party A's now "democratically" imposed call for the use of party B's resources. The compliance siphons both the liberty and resources of B without creating any new resources. This zero-sum game inevitably erodes some of the current resources—rendering it in fact a negative-sum game—by applying them to enforcement rather than to provision of services. Carried to its extreme, it becomes a perpetual and endless game between A and C, draining resources from B until those resources have all been transferred. Then someone must go out to create new wealth to continue feeding this indefatigable system. The final outcome is the relentless expansion of C's power and wealth, while both A and B lose liberties. This power model may be concisely described as a democratically imposed, slow-motion tyranny. Parties A and B lose liberties to party C.

We have begun to view the enforcement of power by an adversary or rival (who, supposedly, have everyone's best interests in mind) as the correct way to do things and, in some cases, the only way to achieve progress. We have apparently come to believe that political might makes right, and we act accordingly. This mindset stands contrary to the traditional concepts of health care, from Hippocrates to modern medicine. Up until the latter half of the twentieth century, patients and medical practitioners expected health care to be rendered in an atmosphere of cooperation. Slavery constituted an exception, an aberration. Mutual caring and healing relationships represent the highest ideals and values of health care. Personalization, responsiveness, and collaboration nourish the relationship, forming trust and an alliance between patient and practitioner.

In stark contrast to this mindset, today's environment is based on the competitive adversarial model of A versus B, which brandishes its legal sword, severs bonds before they can begin, slashes trust asunder, and hacks the potential for mutual respect into shards of suspicion. Typical rhetoric includes calls for compliance with the threat, "Do the right thing, or else," amid the almost plaintive cry, "I know my rights."

Power Costs: Medicare and Medicaid

The inequitable and unjust application of resources represents another significant issue concerning the current health care delivery system, a moral issue most dramatically seen in Medicare and Social Security for citizens over the age of 65. The myth that Medicare represents a social insurance policy has been exploded. There are no financial reserves, no trust funds, and no contracts other than the political guarantee Congress provides from year to year that current income will be paid to seniors, regardless of their financial status.

The moral dilemma arises because citizens over 65 today hold more than an estimated 75% of the private equity of this country. Why should Medicare and Social Security transfer the wealth and wealth equivalents of the financially weakest segments of society to the wealthiest? The moral argument for this transfer of resources from the relatively poor to the relatively rich is tenuous at best. It appears justified only on the basis of political activism and the blunt application of political power.

Originally established to benefit mothers and children, Medicaid programs have deviated from their original intention. In the state of Texas, for example, spending on adults consumes about 74% of Medicaid funds with a substantial proportion allotted to housing senior citizens in nursing homes (Texas Medicaid Program). Other states also divert funds from programs designed to assist poor children, for example, the State Children's Health Insurance Program (SCHIP). In 2005, "87% of Minnesota's SCHIP enrollees were adults, as were 66% of those enrolled in Wisconsin's program. In Arizona—which has one of the highest rates of uninsured children in the nation—56% of those enrolled in SCHIP were adults." (Turner 2007, A8). Moreover, in Medicaid, private HMOs are taking a big and lucrative role in managing care for the poor (Martinez 2006, A1). This diversion of the Medicare and Medicaid programs enriches politically strong seniors while neglecting politically weak children and families at their most economically vulnerable status. Given the demographics of the Baby Boomers, the ticking time bomb is about to explode.

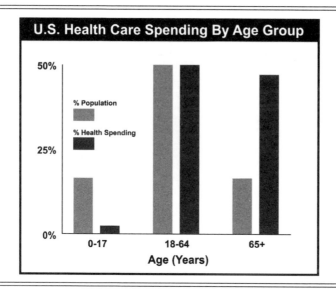

FIG. 3.1

Health Care Benefit Age Profiles

Ratio of Average Spending on Individuals in Each Age Group
Relative to an Individual Age 50-64

Country	0-14	15-19	20-49	50-64	65-69	70-74	75-79	80+
Australia	0.60	0.57	0.64	1.00	1.81	2.16	3.90	4.23
Austria	0.28	0.28	0.46	1.00	1.42	1.75	1.98	2.17
Canada	0.43	0.61	0.65	1.00	2.45	2.44	4.97	7.54
Germany	0.48	0.43	0.58	1.00	1.52	1.80	2.11	2.48
Japan	0.44	0.22	0.43	1.00	1.70	2.20	2.76	3.53
Norway	0.57	0.34	0.52	1.00	1.70	2.21	2.69	3.41
Spain	0.57	0.39	0.48	1.00	1.50	1.50	1.96	1.99
Sweden	0.43	0.43	0.63	1.00	1.50.	1.50	1.96	1.99
United Kingdom	1.08	0.65	0.76	1.00	2.07	2.07	3.67	4.65
United States	0.88	0.82	0.77	1.00	5.01	5.02	8.52	11.53

Fig. 3.2 Source: Kotlikoff, Laurence and Christian Hagist. 2005, December. Who's Going Broke? National Bureau of Economic Research, Working Paper No. 11833, 25.

Power Meets Ethics

Currently, we have neither morally just nor economically value-added approaches to health care spending. Economic and political power dominates principle, exploiting ethics which become a gadget to be tinkered with at the whim of the powerful, rather than a unifying concept that power serves. Some use the phrase "ethical practice" to seize the moral high ground to rationalize their power plays, often scrambling madly and stepping over others to grasp it.

In sectors of the economy other than health care, the provider and the consumer in collaboration determine reasonableness of the cost of a service. If the consumer considers the benefit of the service valuable enough to justify the charge, the agreement between them establishes the charge as reasonable and the provider receives payment accordingly. If not, the consumer either does without the service or looks for it elsewhere.

Recently, the medical director of an insurance company labeled an ongoing dispute with a group of physician providers who had decided not to see patients covered by one of their insurance plans as an "ethical dilemma." The providers based their decision on the fact that services rendered by the providers were often either reimbursed at a small fraction of the charge for the service or denied reimbursement altogether. The administrative burdens of attempting to serve the so-called beneficiaries of this health plan had become too costly for the doctors to provide care to these patients. The insurance company argued that the physicians' charges or services were unreasonable. The dispute concerned who should be the one to determine whether a charge or service is reasonable and the basis on which the determination should be made. It could be the person rendering the service, the person receiving the benefit of the service, or a third party with no part in rendering the service or receiving the health benefit who stood to gain financial profit by acting as an intermediary.

The insurance company, a third party with no hand in either giving or receiving the service, made a unilateral determination that either the services or the charges were unreasonable. Is the determination morally sound? The recipient of the medical service has paid the insurance company funds in the form of premium payments. The insurance company gets to keep as profit funds that it does not have to pay to providers. Thus, whatever the insurance company brands as "unreasonable" or "non-customary" services or charges represents money that it gets to keep as profit. Is this beginning to sound suspiciously like slow-motion tyranny?

The medical director attempted to take the moral high ground by designating the above scenario as an ethical problem generated by the providers' refusal to see the patients. In reality, the providers withdrew from doing business with the insurance company because the providers rendered services they considered necessary at charges they considered reasonable. But the insurance company failed to reimburse the provider by the insurance plan. The patients wanted services from this particular group of providers and deemed them necessary, expressing this by numerous complaints to the insurance company. But the insurance company, holding money that patients had given them, decided the services and charges were inappropriate.

The insurance company finally offered to pay the doctors their billed, rather than discounted, charges. The doctors declined, based on their experience with the insurance company. The medical director then portrayed the doctors as morally deficient—an ethical dilemma, no doubt, but whose behavior initiated the conflict in values? This example is one of countless examples of power dominating principle and of ethics being used as an abstract or business lever rather than as a guiding code in medicine.

Who is so wise and so secure in his own virtue that he should make decisions about what services are appropriate for other individuals? Only in a world that assumes there must be restrictive, rationing choices and that there should be a collective process to make them would such a question be answerable.

We can visualize contrasting strategies—ethical values versus legal constraints—by imagining ethical values as a thick blue arrow contrasting with the thin red lines of legal, bureaucratic, and administrative, power-based regulations.

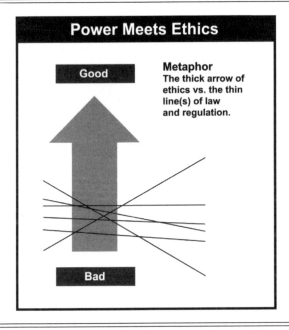

FIG. 3.3

The thick blue arrow represents a continuous process of dynamic improvement in patient-centered medical care. It mirrors history, appreciating the benefits of behaving in ways that are fair, reasonable, and beneficial to society as a whole by first serving individual patients. On the other hand, the thin "red" lines represent externally applied, minimally acceptable standards. These superficial boundary lines invite people to approach minimum standards of conduct rather than to aspire to overall excellence. And after a time, a stance at these base levels starts to be misinterpreted as a gold standard, when it is really a position of minimal competence, principle, and quality. These minimum standards encourage individuals not only to seek the lowest possible common denominator but also to translate this barely acceptable minimum standard into a global goal.

Determining where the minimal red line will be and staying just above it is a waste of energy. Is this lowest common denominator approach really what we want for our health care system, or do we want our doctors and nurses to aspire to be the very best and deliver the most value to patients?

Avoidable Ailments: The Mirror

When analyzing health and health care problems, we must explore all contributing factors including our own behaviors. Another troublesome and questionable allocation of health care resources rests in the huge block of funds spent to treat diseases that could have been avoided by prevention strategies and individual, responsible behavior. With our society focused on the politics of patients' rights and negligence of health care practitioners, we tend toward adversarial enforcement. We fail to ask two hard, basic, utilitarian questions: Do I have the right to live negligently and then demand that someone else pay for resolutions to my resulting ill health? Do I, as a patient, have an obligation to consider my contribution to my own problems? Unpleasant as the task may be, ask yourself the question, "How did I contribute to the problem?"

Why do we find admitting our own contribution so difficult when a problem occurs? The answer to this question is complex. As children, we almost all behave as if we are the center of the universe. We eventually learn that we are not, but we are often more disposed to rationalization, transference, anger, and blaming others for our problems.

Assigning Our Problems to Someone Else

On a grander scale, these same tendencies exist in society and become part of our culture. Just as fear and anger are commonly experienced emotions in individuals, society as a whole also experiences them. And just as these emotions require modulation by higher brain functions in individuals, they do also in society at large, or else they negatively influence behavior to the point of harm to self or others. Unfortunately, driven by immature attitudes, we may let childish methods of dealing with these emotions override more reasonable methods of higher brain function.

Transference, the tendency to reassign a problem to someone else rather than dealing with it ourselves, permeates individuals, societies, and our health care system. The person who transfers a problem to another becomes dependent on the party who is the recipient of the problem.

In individuals, another way of handling a problem is to internalize it. In this case, a person puts the problem in an internal box and builds a wall around it rather than addressing it or finding constructive ways to resolve and manage it. Such a self-created dilemma immobilizes a person and makes him or her feel powerless against the problem. In such a state, alternative solutions presented in the form of legal or bureaucratic intervention often sound very attractive. Presenting the intervention as rescuing the dependent one is common: "This is not your fault. You are a victim; you need someone to take these burdens from you. You have a right to be free of these cares and woes; we will protect and care for you." Individuals often eagerly turn over the problem to the intervening party. The "victim" does not deal with the original problem and creates an additional dependency on someone else who cannot manage it, thereby only adding a manipulating intermediary.

About 60 years ago, the concept of health care entitlement accelerated when wage and price controls arose in the post-World War II economy. Health care evolved into an employment benefit that, once negotiated, became a perceived right. From the early 1960s to today, commercial insurance carriers, in alliance with employers and government, have used marketing and other strategies to position themselves as intermediaries. They sell people on the idea that those who can afford it are entitled to health insurance coverage, that those who cannot may also be entitled, and that the intermediaries process those transactions happily for a government-provided fee. In 1965, Congress cemented the idea of entitlement to health care with the enactment of Medicare and Medicaid. Additional laws, including the Emergency Medical Treatment and Active Labor Act (EMTALA), the Health Insurance Portability and Accountability Act (HIPAA), and the Medicare Modernization Act (MMA), also contributed to the sense that health and health care are inalienable rights on a par with the rights stated in our Constitution.

Our failure to look in the mirror to see our own contributions to our health status and to assume responsibility for those consequences contributes to the culture of entitlement. Political interference leads to health care entitlement claims based on political rights. Over time, and with the collective agreement of the group, this process of turning our problems over to others begins to seem reasonable. What is worse, this dependence on others has been rationalized as necessary. People say to themselves, "I did not create this problem, and I cannot solve it, so I must be the victim of the problem. If I am the victim, then someone must be to blame for it."

As a consequence, we assume a new social status, a formal category of victimhood. This social status becomes politicized and, in the process, wrapped up in a "moral" blanket. Victimhood becomes a basis for a claim of entitlement on the resources of others. People say to themselves, "After all, those at fault should pay." The cultural loop is closed by widespread acceptance of this victimhood status as true and correct, and it becomes cemented in the political culture as entitled rights. Fear and anger lead directly to victimhood, followed by entitled rights.

Turning our problems over to others may feel rational at the time, but when we examine this process, we see that we are making ourselves less powerful, not more so. A person wins and loses at the same time in this bargain. He obtains a promise of help in exchange for liberties and opportunities for self-determination. At some crossroads, people must come to deal with certain realities consciously. They must face their childish and primitive tendencies to blame and let others be responsible for their problems. Our higher brain function has a purpose. It can be used to train, educate, parent, and exert control over basic emotional reactions in order to implement health care solutions. Our health and medical challenges are our problems. Like it or not, we own them. We may ask for and receive help with them, but they are still our problems.

Quality of Life and Length of Life

A lifetime of effort may be required to meet a standard of responsibility sufficient to do two things: maintain your health at optimum levels and preserve the freedom you cherish. While one person's concept of responsibility may meet another's definition of irresponsibility, a useful operating health care standard could be the degree to which behaviors contribute to the two core outcomes: quality of life and length of life.

To the degree that our egocentric ignorance, deficiencies of character, and destructive behaviors result in decreased quality of life and longevity, there will be adverse economic consequences, and investments will yield negative returns. Prudence dictates that a beneficial system should have incentives for healthy behaviors and disincentives for unhealthy ones. Disincentives will likely have an economic component and a social stigma component. In no instance should the system provide economic rewards for bad behavior, a characteristic of our current system. Consider health care, and the people who provide it, to be your best, even most wonderful, friend. You are much more likely to evoke a caring and healing response if you care as well—especially for and about yourself and for and about your relationship with them.

Consequences of Bad Behavior

Ask yourself how your standard of conduct fits with a useful, general standard—the Golden Rule—and what will be the consequences for your life. If you indiscriminately treat others as if they have done you some wrong and that you are their victim, you are diminished. That is not necessarily their fault.

If you choose to be irresponsible, there will be consequences to your behaviors. Despite any notions you may have to the contrary, you become a burden to others. That will cause you to evoke reactions, some charitable, but mostly negative. In turn, you may feel victimized, or strike back in some destructive way. A chain of reactions will occur, some to attempt to coddle you into compliance with the norms of society, others to restrict your liberty and means. Nobody wins, least of all you.

There is no plain and simple way to explain the negativity you create. Your ignorance is no excuse. Your character deficiency is not a disease; it is your failure to assume responsibility for your own actions. Destroying yourself, or destroying others, is never an appropriate behavior because you are not the center of the universe, nor a victim, but merely who and what you are. The first person who can change something that needs to change is you, and after that, everyone else follows. There are many who would help you, but they are not a stage on which you can act out your problems. If you fail to change, there can be no "virtuous" outcomes that will matter to you, your family, or our shared society. Adhering to destructive behaviors and habits only contributes to an unhealthy draining of health care resources, creating a dependence akin to "slave medicine."

References

Martinez, Barbara. 2006, November 15. "Health-Care Goldmines: Middlemen Strike It Rich." *Wall Street Journal*. A1.

Texas Medicaid Program: Medical Information System (MSIS).

Turner, Grace-Marie. 2007, March 17-18. "Insurance Folly." *Wall Street Journal*. A8.

Zakaria, Fareed 2004. *The Future of Freedom*: Illiberal Democracy at Home and Abroad. New York: W. W. Norton and Company.

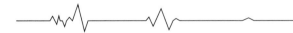

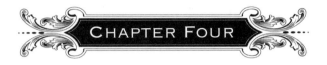

CHAPTER FOUR

Slave Medicine

The floggings will continue until morale improves!

—The New Yorker—

Enslavement by Default

Modern models of entitlement, insurance, managed care, legal protection, and regulatory requirements have led to the unintended, yet inevitable, consequence of the loss of personal liberty. Democracies tend to degrade as voters appropriate the resources of others through the state. They trade their responsibility and their liberty, typically through the vote, for the proverbial sack of silver.

In health care today, we create waste by failing to follow the money, by viewing medicine as a cost center, by the dominance of power-based systems over principle, and by our failure to see in ourselves the causes and solutions of our problems. In a society, these problems transfer to others, who in turn then must solve them. Society is not some third party; it is comprised of each and every one of us. We must act responsibly. If we were alone in the wilderness, most of the societal mores we hold onto so tightly would be moot. We could be afraid or angry, but notions of "victimhood," "entitlement," and "rights" would have no place. The bear, the mountain lion, and the buzzard do not care about the core values that are vital in a human society. When we place those values within the context of society, rationalize our cares and woes, blame others for our problems, or turn to others to solve our problems, we go astray. We run the risk of abandoning or trading our liberties for some notion of safety or security; all the while enslaving ourselves and fellow citizens. Health care today illustrates this sobering dynamic.

Reading the more than 50,000 pages of Medicare's rules and regulations, or any managed-care physician's contract, you will be repelled and chilled at the model of medical care that portends your future. This model hardly benefits free men, but rather more resembles slave medicine dispensed by slave doctors. In the long run, many people will not tolerate this. The key questions remain: What must we endure in the meantime? What looms immediately ahead that can be avoided?

The example from chapter 1, where readers were asked to vote to make doctors into either public servants or independent professionals, rationalizes and calls for a so-called single-payer system. Is this the only type of health care service that should be available? Would those with the means seek private care outside the system? Would seeking private care be legal? These choices concern whether the "slave medicine" would be part-time with doctors doing "government work" on "slave patients" for eight hours and then seeing so-called "free men and women" in private practice for the remainder of their time, or whether "slave medicine" would be full-time, with no option for private care. The latter would represent "slave medicine" all the time for all parties.

The consequences of "slave medicine" are not just personal. There are two additional consequences to consider: waste and demoralization.

Waste and the "Law of Diminishing Returns"

Waste in the current system expands and intensifies despite regulators' efforts to "squeeze the fat out" of the system, and the fix is often worse than the original problem. We are beyond the point of cutting fat; for some, we have advanced now into cutting muscle and moved dangerously close to vital organs.

This waste includes costs and burdens of non-value-added medicine from largely unproven practices and procedures. They include non-value-added processes and procedures imposed from over-regulation and bureaucracy. They include institutionalized inefficiency, both regulatory and financial. Waste occurs also as a by-product of policing the system. Adversarial conflict creates huge costs among patients, care givers, and third parties as they engage in the conflicts of enforcement and plunder, wasting both energy and resources. The negativity of bad behaviors—power-mastery, profiteering, and parasitism—accumulates into a psychological waste heap eroding trust in the system.

We can do—and have yet to do—more about what is unknown and misapplied in medical practice. We must continue the traditional disciplines of medicine, including patient care, research, and education. Evidence-based medicine describes circumstances where evidence demonstrates the benefits derived. This evidence usually results from controlled, masked studies. Much of current medical practice does not have such supporting evidence. Practices have simply accumulated through time, tradition, and experience. We do not know for a fact that all improvements in health status are the result of a particular intervention or whether other treatments may be more effective. There is pervasive uncertainty in the context of the practice of medicine that will not be soon dispelled. Although these factors probably partly contribute to the waste of resources, there is no way to find out without additional research. Unfortunately, resources that could be used to answer these questions are being diverted to other, more wasteful processes.

Substantial concerns persist that medicine does not provide optimal care to many in America, either by doing too much or too little. Maggie Mahar collected detailed evidence on both sides of the equation. The health care marketplace deviates from the "Universal Curve of the Economist," also called the "Law of Diminishing Returns."

The following graphic represents how these forces might apply to and be measured in health care. The value relationship curve depicts the "universal" relationship between the steadily increasing investment of resources or costs and the quality of derivative effects. Within a given enterprise, there will likely be a family of domain curves, each reflecting the incremental effects of resource application. Ideally, these curves should be superimposed upon one another, with minimal internal variation. In fact, there may be significant differences between, for example, investments in people versus information systems. This may reflect either a specific management challenge or a fundamental misalignment between the mission, capacities, products, services, interests, and applications of resources. Variation can be considered major internal evidence of the compromised quality of the aggregate enterprise.

The criteria for the appraisal of value include and go beyond traditional financial measures. In figure 4.1, a graphical approach may be employed to derive a comprehensive view of the functional, value-based health of an enterprise and the risks to it. The results may be applied against a standard represented by a graphical display of quality compared to resources applied. The first measurement may set the baseline for a comparison of subsequent evaluations, or known, external performance standards. In this manner, trends of value, variation in value subsets by activity, indications for management interventions, and the effects of management interventions may be discerned.

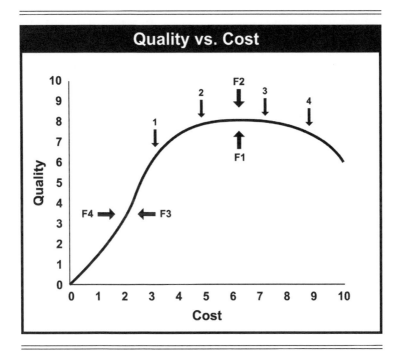

FIG. 4.1 UNIVERSAL CURVE OF THE ECONOMIST LAW
OF DIMINISHING RETURNS

There are three phases in the value curve:

1. Rapidly increasing quality as resources are applied.

2. A plateau, where more resources do not materially improve quality.

3. Decline, where excessive resources cause degradation of effects.

Point 1 could indicate an optimal point for low-cost, acceptable quality practice. A slight decrease in resources may result in rapidly declining quality. Point 2 indicates the optimal point with maximal value derived for costs incurred. Point 3 represents a point of low risk, where increasing or decreasing resources within the range between points 2 and 4 will not cause material deterioration in quality. The diminished risk comes at a cost of wasted resources or the difference in cost between points 2 and 3. Point 4 represents the place where maximum resources are applied to achieve high quality, which also suggests low efficiency. Further application of resources runs the risk of deteriorating quality. The broad arrow labeled F1 indicates the forces and benefits of continuous quality improvement. The broad arrow labeled F2 indicates the forces and burdens of an inevitable, steady degradation of quality. The broad arrow labeled F3 indicates the forces and benefits of efficiency, or decreased cost without diminished quality. The broad arrow labeled F4 indicates the forces and burdens of decreased efficiency, or increased cost without improvement in quality. Forces F1 and F3 increase value, while forces F2 and F4 decrease value.

Non-value-added procedures add excessive regulations and "payer dances" to medical practice. Rules and regulations are internally inconsistent and open to multiple interpretations, useful for providing power and gainful employment to the keepers of the rules but both burdensome and threatening to providers of health care services. Total compliance constitutes a full-time job, in which nothing useful can be obtained. One can do one's best and only hope the enforcers do not need another head on a stake today. Be assured, however, that any time an enforcement agency wants to shut down a given health care enterprise, it can do so under the cover of some rule or regulation.

The "payer dances" have fewer legal risks, but they contain financial risks to patients and to their providers. Payers receive premiums or taxes. In the for-profit world, their job requires them to keep as much of this money as possible so that they and their investors may be as well paid as possible. In politics, the rewards to be obtained are political votes in exchange for promises calculated to either retain votes or get new votes. With this money comes power to achieve sequestered and preferred insurance regulatory protection; power to market to the public and expand their revenue; and power to engage in profitable business practices that retain as much money from the so-called "beneficiaries" as possible. It helps their cause to make the administrative processes so complex that patients and physicians have difficulty conforming. When the payer denies payment, blaming the patients or physicians is a typical fallback position. The net effect of this power transfer to the intermediaries erodes providers' and beneficiaries' liberties and their trust.

Rules and regulations have other unintended consequences. Predators patrol the system, looking for infractions from which they can prosper. In the case of an overzealous enforcement agent, job security, or an opportunity for career advancement, may be at stake. For others, like trial lawyers, the motivation appears more basic: a lottery opportunity. As a consequence, practitioners expend vital energy looking over their shoulders, practicing defensive medicine, paying excessive insurance premiums, or simply withholding a service. If evidence existed to show that these practices enhance the quality of medical services, they might be justifiable. But such evidence does not exist.

Stakeholders: Gatekeepers to the System

An analysis of the reasons health care has become so overtly political reveals the perception that somehow there must be many legitimate stakeholders—a shameless play on the word "shareholders," as if they "own" the system in ways that entitle them to profit. The list moves, in order of the current power and influence in health care, from government legislators, rule-makers, bureaucrats, and enforcement agents at the top, to insurance companies, pharmaceutical companies, and those in the legal system. Finally, the list ends with the hospitals, doctors, and nurses. Patients rank low on the totem pole, largely as a result of the power others hold over them and their limited access to the system. Intermediaries act literally like massive bouncers at popular dance clubs; they are the gatekeepers to the system.

The nature of these stakeholders' "holdings" in the system must be closely examined. Their positions in the system follow a set of assumptions culled from the meaning of the word "stake." If the meaning represents a type of property right, then does this claim rest only on the physical and economic presence of the party, regardless of the value they add to patient care? If so, then the stake may become like a spear or club used to enforce the claim through the threat of injury or pain—if the system does not capitulate to the interests of the stakeholder. If the stake is threatened, enforcement of those interests—money, political, legal, or regulatory power—is sure to follow. The burden can be calculated, but the benefit is doubtful, at least at the level of actual health improvement.

Contrast an adversarial model for health care services with a cooperative model. If the relationships between patients and care providers are cooperative, there will be dialogue, like when friends and family care for one another. In this model, the physician will have in his capacity and role special burdens to do the right thing, and to do it well. The patients will have reciprocal responsibilities to be responsible, active partners and to share in their own care.

Third parties often derive their power from their ability to prosper from conflict. In the adversarial model, you win, I lose, and the third parties, who managed and fostered the conflict, share and even dominate the spoils. In fact, the zero-sum of the game only shifts the resources away from the care process. Accordingly, both patients and doctors lose energy and liberty and third parties win power and money. It is easy to see the better of the two, but we are now systematically voting for the adversarial model, and with this model, the power brokers in the middle are the clear winners.

The following example illustrates how all of this complexity plays out in the current marketplace with multiple stakeholders. Imagine a group of providers eager to participate in a managed care plan that represents the employees of a large company. The plan wishes to attract employees to participate, but only at a price that satisfies their needs and those of their shareholders. The company hires a surrogate to negotiate with providers on behalf of its employees. These surrogates negotiate with an underwriter, or so-called risk taker. That negotiator bargains with a benefits administrator for the company, and, in turn, bargains with an administrative benefits broker. More or less the same sequence occurs on the provider side. The benefits broker negotiates with the provider system broker, who negotiates with the provider system administrator, who negotiates on behalf of the provider system, and then, in turn, bargains with a primary care gatekeeper, who may approve referral to a specialist. On both sides, each level has its own set of tools and rules. This maze of bureaucracy is what currently separates patients and their providers. This system wastes money, and this process also suggests that patients and doctors are neither capable nor trustworthy to develop their own relationship—in the context of the current political culture—and therefore not free to relate directly.

If we were to spend our resources on actual patient care while providing transparent information to the public about how the money is being spent for the actual outcomes achieved, there would be more than enough money to afford to do the right things in prevention, education, research, and patient care. However, this outcome can happen only if we will simply stop wasting time, energy, and money on non-value-added processes (NVAPs), non-value-added medicine (NVAM), and the consequences of individual bad behavior.

Demoralization: Degradation of Human Potential

Current health care practices exhibit a more tragic and ultimately threatening trend than economic waste. When values become skewed and wealth matters more than the quality of human interaction, all parties suffer. The degradation of human potential occurs through demoralization. One might conclude that degradation and demoralization are inevitable, given the human propensity to make promises we cannot keep and to punish others for our own bad judgment. Folk wisdom shows that good judgment comes from experience, but unfortunately, experience comes from bad judgment. We cannot be freed from the web we weave, but we must directly face the fact that demoralization persists in both patient and physician communities.

Power-based structures and processes use fear and anger to draw patients ultimately to accept the "design" of our current health care system. Seething emotions proliferate when problems fail to be resolved and a pervasive, angry feeling persists. Surveys demonstrate that vast majority of Americans are angry about one or several problems with the health care system; very few of them acknowledge any responsibility for its circumstances.

Power structures seize the situation and reinforce it with rhetoric and promises that cannot be kept. Now, even the so-called "beneficiaries" see the reality of the bad situation. Seniors believe they will "get theirs" but know that others who follow them will not receive the same benefits that they have come to enjoy. Politicians know, yet will not touch the "third rails" of Social Security and Medicare. Meanwhile, the power enforcers, profiteering intermediaries, and predatory and parasitic packs work within the current "red-line" rules of the system to get whatever can be picked off. The system mirrors ecosystem life itself, passing from bountiful to barren. The outcome looks inevitable and there is little question about how the game will end. The only question to be resolved is whether the end will be cataclysmic, or if the current, prolonged agony will end with nothing more than a calculable date of bankruptcy. Most seniors know what will happen to their grandchildren, even as they turn a blind eye to the situation themselves.

On the physician side, the story looks equally tragic. About two decades ago, a cartoon in *The New Yorker* depicted an ancient galley ship powered by slave oarsmen. One of the oarsmen was being whipped while he was tied to the mast. "The floggings will continue until morale improves!" announced the slave master in the caption. This notion has penetrated modern culture in a number of ways and one of those is the manner in which society has chosen to use physicians. This dynamic is not unprecedented, and it has at least a forty-year history.

Physicians are not alone in being treated in this way. There has been a progressive depreciation of the value of the sacrifices made by health care providers to become what they are and to sustain their commitment to health care. The debts they owe for their long and expensive education and the delayed gratification they receive, seem irrelevant to the champions of our national treasury. Good and experienced providers leave the profession.

"This is not what I signed up for; I don't need this, and I'm out of here," say young and idealistic physicians.

Some become jaded and depressed, saying: "If this is the way I am to be treated, so be it; they will get what they deserve."

Perhaps worst of all, the brightest, most talented, and prospective physician candidates say, "My doctor friends and parents tell me not to do what they do; they say I should go into some other profession such as law or business. It's much less risky, and I am more likely to be able to support my family that way." Meanwhile, doctors in the middle of their careers feel trapped.

Five stages of enterprise health deterioration have been observed as following a progression: success, subsistence, stress, shock, and shut-down. Most physicians huddle somewhere in the middle, under stress, with an increasing number in a state of professional shock. To the degree that forces keep increasing the heat on the health care pot, all of us will suffer consequences. The present condition of health care is not safe for anyone, especially patients. We must develop a solution that provides high quality patient care, adequately compensates health care providers for their dedication to excellence in the profession, and attracts our best and brightest minds.

References

Mahar, Maggie. 2006. *Money-Driven Medicine*. New York: Harper Collins. (Chapters 1-5 are especially relevant).

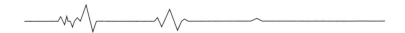

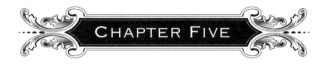

CHAPTER FIVE

Lurching toward Solutions

God bless the Americans. They can always be counted on to do the right thing . . . but only after they've tried everything else.

—Winston Churchill—

Inappropriate Shepherd of Health Care

The Sherman Antitrust Act of 1890 created the legal justification for the regulation of health care in America. The Supreme Court later made additional rulings subjecting the "learned professions," including medicine, to the jurisdiction of the Federal Trade Commission (FTC). Primary regulatory and enforcement authority for the Sherman Antitrust Act belongs to the Federal Trade Commission. These laws and decisions were passed in the name of promoting competition to stimulate the provision of services at the lowest market price possible. These policies and decisions date to the mid 1970s and were reaffirmed in U.S. Supreme Court decisions (Goldfarb 1975 and Bates 1977).

Additional enforcement also emanates from Inspectors General at the Justice Department, the Health Care Financing Administration, the Federal Trade Commission, and state authorities. Overlapping boundaries make authority frequently unclear in health care. The regulatory menu is long, including numerous unfunded mandates, culminating in the complex Medicare Modernization Act of 2003. Maggie Mahar called this act a "last ditch" effort to privatize health care (Mahar, 325).

All these laws, court decisions, and administrative rulings resound with a single clear message. Official government policy declares medicine and medical care to be an industry with a fundamentally commercial nature; medicine and medical care is subject to the Sherman Antitrust Act. This policy almost certainly is wrong; the "industry" has never been responsive as a true market. The cost of the effort to enforce the general will of society with legions of lawyers and bureaucrats and the consequential loss of innovation and productivity have been and promise to be intolerably high. What is further incalculable is the loss of trust among the parties. In the 1960s, a common phrase was "Don't trust anybody over thirty." In the 2000s, it has been replaced with "Don't trust anybody." Because of this loss of trust, we have punished everybody, including ourselves.

The Federal Trade Commission is an inappropriate shepherd for health care in our culture. Its reason for being, its assumptions about the nature of the world, and its methods for addressing perceived problems run counter to the best interests of patient care. Health care is not about commerce; it's about caring and healing.

Aligning Finance, Culture, and Incentives

The following graphic shows a view of the interaction of health care, politics, and economics in our culture. The central contention argues that culture rules. The red arrows in the diagram depict the flow of influence.

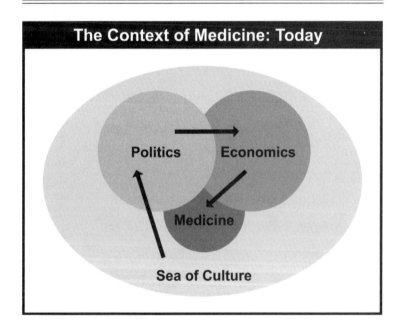

FIG. 5.1

The graphic clarifies how society's efforts and resources should ideally be focused. The influence of culture cannot be overstated. In democracies, culture directly rules politics. In other forms of government, it enables politics. Politics rule economics and economics rule medicine. It would be fantasy to believe otherwise.

For at least two and a half centuries, political observers have noted that one of the flaws of democracy—a potentially fatal one—is the capability of the population to vote to seize money and redistribute it through the state. This group confiscation, based on amoral self interest, uses the political process that goes with it to cloak itself in moral rhetoric and justification. One example in health care is the Medicare program. Like all government entitlements, it is a so-called "pay-as-you-go" system. From the perspective of a senior beneficiary, the system should be called "you-pay-as-I-go." Neither liberty nor morality has been served in the transfer. There is not a one-size-fits-all modulator for this reality. To rationalize this apparent irregularity without a conflict between generations, or intolerable debt loads to future citizens, presents an intractable challenge. This problem constitutes a major test of our democracy.

The medical provider community faces a looming shortage of physicians. Initial concerns centered on the aging Baby Boomers and the likelihood of a burgeoning demand for physicians. Now we can foresee a potential decline in the quality of U.S. applicants to medical schools and, consequently, the future of health care in America. In about 1970, observant deans of medical schools began to notice a drop in the quantity of applicants and a dip in the quality of applicants. An influx of quality female applicants apparently ameliorated the circumstance. We now run the risk that even our quality women may not make up for the projected diminished capacity of applicants. Too many of the best and brightest go into the study of law and business—bad news for medicine, bad news for citizens.

Assuming that we have manpower and quality issues to face, there are a number of options. We have tried, mostly by squeezing, to get physicians to work harder, and in response, they have. Now that option is about played out, particularly for experienced physicians who have other options, including early retirement. We could mandate the training of more physicians, but that is very expensive. That would not improve quality and in fact may do the opposite, and the lead time is long given the rigors of medical education. We do not have the time, even if we had the inclination. We could import physicians from other countries. But that has not solved our problems in the past, and it punishes other countries by draining the brightest minds from their society.

Other ways of dealing with the health care crisis do not present us with attractive solutions. The question of whether quality physicians would want to come to the United States in the future is problematic. We may have a more positive view of ourselves than others do. We could export U.S. citizens to other countries for medical training, but that may not meet expectations for educational quality. We could export care to other countries where it can be purchased more inexpensively. To be sure the trend to seek medical care in less expensive venues continues, for example, as patients seek international options for plastic surgery, transplantation, and virtual services like radiologic interpretations. Additional niche markets have emerged for remote consultative services. The promise of technology to locally dispense medications following inter-continental diagnoses has become reality. Surgery performed robotically by remote surgeons is being explored. *New York Times* columnist and author Tom Friedman correctly notes that in important economic ways, the world truly has become flat (Friedman 2005). All of this has left U.S. physicians in a pickle, and the surrounding culture has been the curing vinegar.

These approaches may fit conceptually into an industrial model for health care where doctors and hospitals are viewed as interchangeable parts in a system controlled by all-knowing and powerful "stakeholders." Such thinking is prevalent among power (i.e., "slave") masters. But that point of view is hard to comprehend and defend given the essence of medical practice and the relationships required for effectiveness.

We are left then with the public perception that health care is too expensive, inefficient, and untrustworthy. The health care system has failed to deal with this perception. As the dangers increase, a patient perceives he or she receives a deteriorating quality of care. Quality, results, and information vary widely. Couple these perception problems with the entitlement culture, and the message our culture concludes is "We deserve better; we live in a land of plenty; I worked hard, and deserve this." It plays out as a terribly conflicted morality play, which it is.

Why has health care brought us to an economic precipice that even Social Security could not? It has to do with financial projections and calculations of net present value. It was a relatively easy matter to know what was going to be required to sustain Social Security. The timeline for pay-out is extended for many years, and the dollars paid were much less in value when seen from the perspective of an individual contributor, who was to become a beneficiary. Hence, the net present value was calculable and worked in the government's favor. If any money had actually been invested at the time it was received by the government, the system might have been sustainable indefinitely.

Medicare and Medicaid have a very different reality with regard to the net present value. Monies need to be spent today against some future possible gains. The gains must be depreciated because the value delivered is received in the future, when the dollars spent have less value. Moreover, there is the unpredictability of persons paying in, which is known with Social Security with respect to age, projected life span, and future benefits. Compare this financial reality to unpredictable medical events of health care that must be paid for today, generally without question or limit. We know better than to say there is no value. Finance, culture, and incentives need to be aligned.

Resolution Bases

Up to this point, we have described health care as a paradoxical enterprise operating in the best and worst of times. We have pointed out the powerful stakeholders and interests who control health care, and we have indicated serious problems that result from treating medicine as a "cost center." With this background, we can now begin to formulate a strategy for solutions to health care problems in the best interests of all the parties.

Ethics: Power Must Serve Principle

The first pillar on the foundation of ethics in health care supports moral values. Dynamic quality is the prime moral value in health care. We have tried the power route and it failed because the system is unraveling. The existing models have inherent flaws satisfying no one. A regulated marketplace inevitably evokes the philosophy of buyer beware. A system of third-party enforcers yields a perversion of the traditional principle of liberty to do the right thing without doing anyone any harm. In the end, such systems breed schemes to maximize the extraction of resources, while performing the minimum needed, and receiving the maximum compensation for the services. The financial rules of the profiteers and the regulatory rules of the enforcers actually have become the game. This condition perverts and corrupts the system with the predictable result of greed, graft, and fraud. This is in an intolerable situation in a profession with moral responsibilities. Power must be in service to principle, and principle determinations must be made by the parties to the relationship—patients and caregivers—rather than enforcers.

Delivery Model

The second pillar on the foundation of ethics in health care supports a culture-based, responsive delivery model. A Presidential Commission to Congress in 1983 recommended a preferred model for the delivery of health care, entitled "Doctor-Patient Accommodation." The cycle is predictable: culture drives politics, and politics drives economics; citizens do choose, actively or by default, the kind of society sustained. We are not passive recipients of our own culture; we make it up and make it happen.

Creating an appropriate cultural setting should be founded upon the clinical encounter, the core or central point where all of the derived values from health care services converge. When a doctor and patient come together, generally in a ten-by-twelve foot room, all of the history and administrative processes that preceded and all of the future additional tests and procedures that follow are concentrated in that moment. The interaction of two persons—one with a perceived medical need or purpose and the other with presumed expertise and commitment—work together in the best interest of the patient to solve problems.

In this context, "The enemy is disease" (Berwick 2005). Provided each of the two parties is willing to behave cooperatively toward that interest, there should be little need for enforcers. The advantages of cooperative relationships, as distinct from adversarial ones, cannot be overstated. If disease is the enemy—and it is—then that should be the exclusive focus of the system. The importance of the cultural context is emphasized by Eric Cassell: "Medical care—in all of medicine, not just primary care—is a human interaction between patient and doctor within a context and in a social system. As such it is not a commodity" (Cassell 1997, 381).

"Why would I want to pick a fight with the doctor who is trying to save my life?" asked one cancer patient, in response to a recommendation by a frustrated family member who was demanding more information from a doctor while suggesting that some legal means might be used as a last resort.

To the degree that society has focused on rules and enforcement to achieve its ends in health care, the price has been inordinately high and the cost burden of the effort has been suffocating. The rules set minimum standards for behavior and then invite minimum compliance. The net effect is that an individual focuses on the red lines, conforms behavior to them, and even claims virtue on the basis of adherence to a minimum legal standard and absence of incarceration! This is clearly not the focus of the best and brightest in medicine, nor is it in the enlightened interests of patients. The aspiration should be an approach to the best possible outcome, without the negativity.

A culturally sensitive approach will focus on the cooperative, clinical encounter to maximize both health and wealth. A higher intelligence at work here will minimize the need for regulatory oversight. Compatible doctors and patients will seek each other out. Rules could be limited to the Golden Rule, "Do unto others as you would have them do unto you."

Under these conditions, the next graphic shows a revised way of looking at influences on culture. Principle-based values define medical practice, and they define the most appropriate economic model. Political culture should be receptive to the benefits, and political culture should be influenced in such a way as to support the interests of the body politic and its culture. The negative cycle is thus reversed.

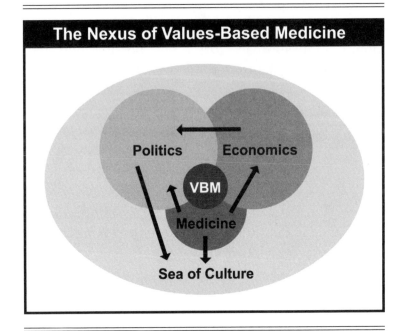

The Nexus of Values-Based Medicine

Politics Economics

VBM

Medicine

Sea of Culture

FIG. 5.2

Our Most Powerful Engine
for Economic Growth

The third foundational pillar supports a cooperative and effective economic model to align the incentives and best interests of doctors and patients. The primary focus should be on an investment in the value of citizens, rather than the cost of caring for them, because the approach is both more business-like and moral. Since you manage what you measure, a central focus should be on metrics, and in turn, those metrics should focus on both human and economic values.

In other words, methods must integrate clinical outcome metrics with economic consequences. These metrics will include clinical quality processes, particularly to the degree that they produce meaningful outcomes. They also will include investment costs and returns to the economy and society.

Time is a critical common factor for each of these. The analysis, therefore, should be amenable to net present value analysis at any time in the value production cycle. For any type of clinical encounter from research through prevention to definitive treatment, the health care system will be able to measure the economic good derived from the patient outcome achieved.

The Lasker Foundation has strongly supported medical research with an emphasis on cardiovascular care. To determine whether these investments in cardiovascular research paid actual dividends, they engaged several schools of economics to assist them in the analysis. From 1970 to 1990, one consequence of improvements in cardiovascular care was a several-year increase in life expectancy. This increase in longevity yielded a direct contribution to the U.S. Gross Domestic Product of about $48 trillion! They reached the conclusion that almost any investment in medical research was highly likely to pay substantial dividends. Couple this with the Nordhaus calculation—that about 50% of the growth in the U.S. economy in the twentieth century was attributable to improvements in health and health care—and we have a basis for an alignment strategy. Health care is our most powerful engine for economic growth. It dwarfs all other growth engines, which only emphasizes the importance of getting this right. We dare not approach health care as a cost center ruled by other sectors of the economy. That sort of thinking is wrong-headed in a society of free individual persons, where the only relevant context for the evaluation of human or economic value relates to them. In fact, improvements in health will provide for much of the growth in other sectors. The abstraction is not health but wealth. Health is the tangible good.

One More Time

Patients and those who support them—principally doctors and nurses—define health care. They represent most of what is necessary and sufficient for health care to occur. Patients, as the center of a principle-driven health care universe, should have both privilege and responsibility. Most people understand the value of health and of health care, yet other worldly considerations intrude and limited resources dictate short-term choices. Now that the entitlement structure has achieved such an enormous proportion, the reasonable fear exists that the failure to provide health care services will create civil unrest and an additional demand backed by threats of disobedience. We can only wonder what will happen if we continue to purchase social tranquility with unfulfilled promises of medical goods and services provided by a shrinking bank of others' resources. It's not difficult to foresee a time when health care may become so scarce that its remaining providers require police protection, and patients may have to endure the rationing of services through physical enforcement.

Social tranquility purchased in exchange for quality health care, particularly if maintained by physical force, represents lost liberty. The notion that we might suppress aberrant and aggressive social behaviors with cash equivalent health services represents a capitulation to a cycle of ever-increasing demands for "protection." It is the political and business equivalent of a racket and health care providers intensely dislike it. Witness the two New York hospitals that have filed a racketeering lawsuit against UnitedHealth Group and several of its affiliates. They contend that the health insurance business is a racket, literally (Krugman A13). Personal responsibility will be required to change the culture that sustains this reality. An American population "bristling with rights" has contributed to our "risk-free, cost-free" assumptions. If we are to be free, we must work collaboratively. We do not have the option to waste our efforts on non-value-added structures or processes.

Today, doctors and nurses enter into medicine with a values-laden set of expectations for themselves. They have been placed under duress. I do not mean to suggest that physicians and nurses are in a unique position with regard to the "boiling pot" of contemporary society. I only pose the idea that we all are paying an inordinately high price for failing to honor the personal investment, sacrifice, commitment, talent, and services of our physicians and nurses more than we currently do.

A resolution can begin with physicians. If you take all the challenges and burdens of becoming a physician and place them on the liability side of a balance sheet, they may be too much to overcome in the current environment. We are not attracting our best and brightest youth in sufficient numbers to our most critical human and economic endeavor. Many still come with the best intentions because there is a caring nature within them that will not be denied; something in the practice of medicine feeds their souls. For those who will deserve and receive it, there is no greater gift. On the other hand, we have demonstrated that we too often snuff out some of our brightest lights. We can do so much better with an approach that will reverse most of the negativity.

In the context of a patient with cancer, the disease is not impressed with the regulatory protection of the host, profit margins of insurance companies, or the so-called market based "reforms." No regulator, power broker, administrator, or bureaucrat is likely to care for cancer in times of need or to cure a patient. No insurance plan, executive, or employee can purge a body of its unwelcome invaders. No additional "out of pocket" expense (to avoid "moral hazard"), price list on a doctor's or hospital's window, or health savings account will improve red and white blood cell counts. Soon, the Supreme Court may follow the wisdom of the people and rule that medicine is not an accumulation of commercial transactions that should be subject to the contrary premises and world views of the Sherman Antitrust Act and Federal Trade Commission.

The reasoning behind the love affair with advertising for medical services seems entirely constructed on premises that might be appropriate for aesthetics and sensory pleasures but is inappropriate for the care of a patient with cancer or any other disease.

We Must Change Our Ways

Human interactions define and are defined by relationships. According to this definition, we must decide what kind of relationship patients wish to have with nurses and physicians. Will this relationship be cooperative or adversarial?

None of the current models for health care fits the bill for a cooperative relationship. One approach is to mandate a single-payer system, that is, government-sponsored-and-delivered health care. The second approach is the so-called competitive market-driven model, where consumers have more responsibility to pay and make choices based on price and quality. But there are two core elements left unattended in the marketplace: 1) The important destiny of the relationships between patients and doctors and 2) The end purposes of the activity.

A third approach, exemplified by the state of Massachu-setts, is mandated health insurance for all residents, sup-ported by the state if necessary. This solves the problem of the uninsured but institutionalizes the current challenges of waste and loss of freedom.

Rhetoric about "healthy communities" and "quality of care" is largely promotional, yet the actual practice of medicine is increasingly detached from fundamental, constituent relationships and legitimate ends. The end result of each approach is the same. The system will be dominated by third parties—government, insurance, industry, or, more likely, a coalition. These third parties will consume resources of time, talent, and money that should be applied to patient care and divert it to non-pa-tient care and non-value-added processes that ultimately must enslave both beneficiaries and providers to meet and feed their profit and power needs.

Looking at investment in the health and wealth of our society, we must change our ways. Nothing we can do in any other sphere of our lives will equal the human and economic productive contributions of optimal health and health care. Part II sets out a set of solu-tions and a pathway for their implementation that we can afford to sustain.

References

Berwick, Donald. 2005, December 7. "Kevin speaks." Keynote address, fourth annual National Forum on Quality Improvement in Health Care. Berwick acknowledges that he borrowed the phrase "The competition that matters is against disease" from Dr. Paul Batalden of the Dartmouth Medical School.

Cassell, Eric. 1997. *Doctoring: The Nature of Primary Care Medicine.* New York: Oxford University Press.

Friedman, Tom. 2005. *The World is Flat.* New York: Farrar, Straus, Reese, and Giroux.

Goldfarb v. Arizona State Bar. 1975. Permitted advertising by professionals and included "learned professions"—previously excluded by Parker v. Brown (1943)—and was affirmed by Bates v. Arizona State Bar (1977), thereby reaffirming the purview of the Sherman Antitrust Act and oversight by the Federal Trade Commission, while giving additional encouragement and direction to medical advertising.

Krugman, Paul. 2007, February 26. "System itself is diseased." *Dallas Morning News*, A13.

Mahar, Maggie. 2006. *Money-Driven Medicine.* New York: Random House.

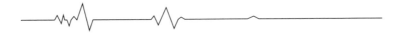

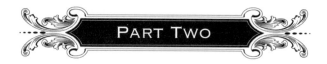

PART TWO

The Solution: Values-Based Medicine

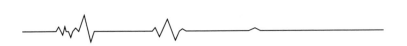

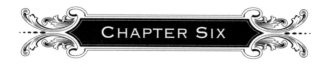

CHAPTER SIX

What's Important

We hold these truths to be self-evident; that all men are created equal; that they are endowed by their creator with certain unalienable rights; that among these are life, liberty, and the pursuit of happiness; that to secure these rights, governments are instituted among men, deriving their just powers from the consent of the governed; that whenever any form of government becomes destructive to these ends, it is the right of the people to alter or to abolish it; and to institute new government, laying its foundation on such principles, and organizing its powers in such form, as to them shall seem most likely to effect their safety and happiness.

—Thomas Jefferson, Declaration of Independence—

The Important Questions

Medicine spans not only the technical aspects of disease and its treatment but also the moral and human dimensions of well-being and illness. Medicine is the most humane of the sciences and the most scientific of the humanities. It's an art as well as a science. Medicine rarely fulfills the quest for "absolute truth." Faculty members of a medical school frequently present to students the ambiguity of medicine's journey, saying, "You will learn many things in the next four years, but there is a problem— half of what you learn will be useful and correct, and the other half will prove wrong. You will spend the rest of your lives trying to figure out which is which."

Practitioners choose a life of discipline and inquiry, constantly testing uncertainties in patient care, education, and research. Society struggles with these same uncertainties when creating policies for the delivery of health care.

Each of us decides how to face our health challenges and how to relate to those who care for us medically. We must first struggle with these questions individually and then establish social policy around the answers.

From the perspective of vigorous good health, humans tend to treat health care as a technical problem with technological and scientific answers, managed by almost mechanical structures and processes. But the best solution to the dilemma of providing health care addresses experientially all the elements of what it means to be human: physically, emotionally, and spiritually.

Only Two Meaningful Outcomes

In health care, there are only two meaningful outcomes—quality and length of life. Living well and living longer are ingrained in our minds and our culture. While understanding and measuring longevity proves easy enough, philosophers wrestle with the specifics of a quality life. Robert Pirsig wrote, "Quality doesn't have to be defined. You understand it without definition, ahead of definition. Quality is a direct experience independent of and prior to intellectual abstractions" (Pirsig 1991, 73).

Pirsig's definition makes irrelevant much of what we currently do in the context of health care quality analysis. Quality ought to be defined by patients, rather than by the limited perspective of a third party, such as an insurance company. The real point where health care becomes defined is in the clinical encounters between patients and caregivers. You know best about the value of your experiences—better than health care advocates, community activists, bureaucrats, company executives, administrators, or politicians. You know what aspects of your life have quality, and you have a reasonable way of balancing what you value. We do not need armies of others defining qualities and values for us. The best way to create a balanced health care environment is to make choices that demonstrate what we value—the quality and length of life.

The means by which we measure quality of life is called "utility analysis." Utility in health care is the quality of life associated with a particular health status. This point will be a prime focus of the framework of solutions to follow.

Resolving Conflicts in Values

In a society, there may be conflicts among what individuals value in life. In a medical context, these differences take on an additional intensity as life itself may be threatened by certain choices, and the intensity of human emotions is raised. Resolution must be reached between individual and societal interests, technical and moral values, static and dynamic mechanisms for quality assurance, and cooperative and adversarial models for quality enhancement.

We must design a system of caring for one another that is moral and we must get the values right in the beginning, middle, and end. If we treat health care as purely technical, or as an industrial or regulatory challenge, we will get it wrong at every turn. We are living right now with that fundamental mistake.

Consider the example of competence in our caregivers. We all hope for competence in those who care for us. We go to some lengths with processes to assure ourselves about their competence, but unfortunately, most of those processes focus on the purely technical aspects of health care rather than on the caregivers' foundation of moral competency.

Today there is a split over what kind of competency is required for effective medical practice. This competency is defined by science, technology, and morality, and it goes well beyond matters of etiquette to the center of the relationship between a doctor and patient. Patients expect kindness from physicians and their associates by the nature of their calling, and physicians deserve the same in return from their patients. Resolving differences can begin with patients and their doctors choosing to be kind to each other. Approaching the complicated issue of providing quality health care with kindness is a great way to begin to fundamentally reform the system.

The study of the ethical and moral implications of discoveries and scientific advances, as in the fields of genetic engineering, provides principles to help us discuss and resolve moral differences concerning the provision of health care. Relevant principles include autonomy, beneficence, non-maleficence, justice, and life. We will discuss each of these important principles in turn.

AUTONOMY

The positive obligation physicians and nurses bear to enhance the personal independence or empowerment of patients creates autonomy. Autonomy occurs through enhancing patient health and improving the patient's capacity for healthy decision-making. Through education, the patient has a greater chance of gaining the good health he or she seeks by making wise choices and avoiding poor ones. The fundamental role of the physician as a patient's teacher is underestimated. The political counterpart of autonomy is liberty, and with liberty comes responsibility.

BENEFICENCE

Being kind, generous, or beneficial characterizes beneficence. It carries the positive obligation of a physician or a nurse to do right things on behalf of patients. This traditional value of medicine has been mischaracterized in our modern world of consumer enlightenment and activism. Kindness and generosity may be mistaken as being overly paternalistic or manipulative and in conflict with autonomy. Physicians and nurses must be trained to discern when autonomy or beneficence should dominate the care and treatment. The patient is usually the ultimate source for making clear what he or she needs.

NON-MALEFICENCE

The medical profession deeply imbues traditional medical practitioners with the admonition, *primum non nocere*, "first do no harm." Non-maleficence means that the care and treatment provided must be intended to better the patient's health and quality of life. This warning does not mean that risky procedures or treatments must be absolutely avoided but that the risks must be fully explained in a way that enables the patient to choose whether or not to undergo a proposed treatment.

JUSTICE

Justice has two components that may at times be in conflict with one another. Individual justice speaks to the correct or just thing to do for individual patients. It implicitly assumes that the greater good will be served by these collected, individual just acts. Distributive justice speaks to the obligations of physicians to seek out a greater good for a group or population. This principle implicitly assumes that more individuals will prosper with good health if the general well-being of the community is served.

The potential for conflicts, particularly as one approaches the interests of individual patients, is obvious. Indeed, entire professional disciplines are organized around such distinctions, such as independent practitioners serving individual patients as distinct from public health or epidemiologic specialists. The issues of justice are intensely focused when the availability and allocation of real resources are considered. Justice is particularly at issue when individuals are denied a medically useful service because they cannot pay for it, or because some other power-based criterion denies them a service.

LIFE

Life and its preservation may be in conflict with the other principles and other points of view in a society. For some, human life is to be cherished to the exclusion of all other considerations. This assumption provides limited room for discussion, and talk about it frequently tends toward the forcing of one particular set of beliefs upon another. There are also challenges in defining what it means to be alive: is a body in a persistent vegetative state "alive"? Some regard cell-based human life, regardless of the systems required for its sustenance, as sufficient to require maintenance. Beliefs about the degree to which one wishes to have life-saving technology applied at the beginning or the end of life are often cherished and not subject to change or debate.

Such beliefs often hinder discussions more than they inform decisions. We must come to some consensus about these issues in order to create quality health care. From a societal perspective these issues become political matters subject to the application of the law. When resolutions are sought by political and legal means alone, they come with a significant cost. They will be driven by culture. To the extent that beliefs about values trump rational analysis, culture is diminished and tends to political enforcement of majority opinion. We likely can do better through informed discourse, a cooperative and collaborative function.

Core Resources: Time, Energy, Dynamic Quality, and Vital Signs

Core resources are the tools available to aid us in creating the most beneficial system of providing health care. They include time, energy, dynamic quality, and vital signs.

TIME

The time we have as living human beings is worthy of special note because all other resources are irrelevant without it. The beginning and end of disease, the timing and duration of medical care, the duration and intensity of side effects, and the application of available resources are all critically dependent on time. Although it is not our only resource, it is our most important one. In human terms, it is relatively easy to measure.

ENERGY

Energy is both characteristic of and an important physical tool for humans. We produce and use physical, intellectual, and emotional energy that directly interacts with and intimately changes our environment and relationships. These changes are for better or worse and for good or bad (positive and negative). Our challenge is purposefully to control and channel these energies for positive outcomes. For physical tasks, most of us recognize good performance or constructive results. We may not fully appreciate how difficult it is to perform at our best, but we do appreciate the results. We intuitively sense how positive emotional energy is created and received when we are loved, supported, and treated kindly.

DYNAMIC QUALITY

The biggest challenge for a good and just society is how to receive and process the highest and best dynamic, intellectual energy available. We struggle with what has merit, what is acceptable, and where we should invest our individual and collective resources. Sometimes it takes a long time, but we have reasonably good, long-term sense. Short-term behaviors, particularly when they are self indulgent or destructive, give us the biggest challenges. The key is to remain open to dynamic innovation and not be consumed by static patterns and structures. Too much regulation or too many rules stifle progress.

Like other energies, money can be used in a positive way for good or in a negative way. In health care, our purpose must be to use money and energy as a means for good. There are no practical limits to the amount of energy available. Our job in health care is to convert energy sources to the highest levels for the good of patients.

VITAL SIGNS

"Vital signs" refers to basic measures of bodily functions, like temperature, pulse, and respiration (TPR). In health care systems, "vital signs" are people, resources, and timing (PRT). The focus should be on creating a positive clinical encounter between a person needing health care and providers with the necessary medical equipment at the earliest possible time to maximize a good result.

A Simple System

Feedback mechanisms are tools of appraisal that reflect the effects of a means applied to achieve intended goals. Correctly chosen, these mechanisms enable a system to be fine-tuned. The following framework provides a structure for meeting goals in the provision of health care.

Means are the resources and methods required to achieve goals. Goals are the objects or results toward which effort is directed. The ends represent the final limit in time and space, the extent of influence, or the range of possibility. When these important ideas are applied to health and the health care system, the framework schematic looks like this:

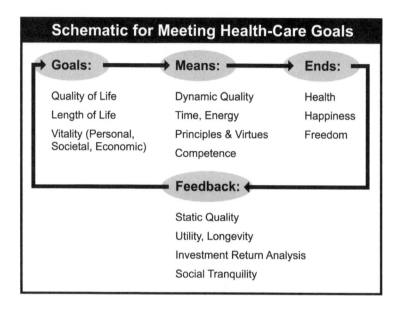

FIG. 6.1 VALUES-BASED MEDICINE: A SIMPLE SYSTEM

Any proposed or enacted health care system should be subject to analysis by the above schematic to ensure that it meets the standard of providing the necessary means to reach the goals and ends.

Threats to Your Health "Business"

The structure of modern health care has been dislodged from its ethical roots. Power and money are holding health care hostage. Despite advances in understanding diseases and the promise of expanding capacities in science and technology, the health care environment is layered with hobbling complexities. This dislocation of modern health care from its roots comes with a great cost. The consequences are waste and misspent resources. So-called "modern" health care constructs like entitlement, insurance, managed care, legal protection, and regulatory requirements have resulted in the restriction of personal liberty. As a result of the current system, our social, economic and medical well-being are at risk. The current system is wasteful because we spend so much on non-value-added processes that invest no discernable benefit to patient care.

Before a health care disaster occurs, a new foundation for a reformed health care system that is workable, effective, and beneficial must be constructed. This foundation should rest upon the following eight supporting design principles:

1. Values, not power, should be the drivers of health care.

2. Two health outcomes—quality of life and longevity—should be our goal.

3. Two jobs—taking care of patients or taking care of someone who is—are the prime contributors to valued health outcomes.

4. Quality of life and longevity drive major subsidiary, economic benefits, and the economic system should be designed to maximize those benefits.

5. Health care is a personal and societal investment that pays huge dividends to society; it is not a cost center.

6. Liberty will not be traded for promises of security that progressively enslaves health care users and providers.

7. Health care will be a collective and individual responsibility with everyone learning to take steps to manage it personally.

8. Health care will be thought of as a long-term family business, with each member prospering or failing together.

Health care is as complex as humanity, but we should not be blinded by that complexity. We must be in charge of our own destinies. To the degree that we opt out, blame others, make demands of others, or seek a protective wing of security, we trade something of our own potential to power-based enforcement structures. The power of these structures depends only on the resources and liberty that we give to them. We must address our future as a cultural, political, and economic society. Happiness, freedom, and wealth are highly dependent on good health.

Our current health care mess is not the work of some-one else. It was caused by our culture, society, values, and actions, as part of our individual and collective consciousness. The following was originally ascribed to W. Edwards Deming and was attributed to the health care context by Donald Berwick, MD, of the Institute of Healthcare Improvement: "Every system is perfectly designed to achieve the results it gets." (Berwick 2005).

If we do not like the results, we must first acknowledge that our own actions and systems achieved them. We can-not blame someone else, claim ourselves to be victims, or depend on others to solve these problems. That someone else may have failed to meet our expectations or con-tributed to our problems is irrelevant because they will always be ours to solve. When we achieve a solution, we become freer. Blaming others is a waste of energy. Freedom and democracy are blessings that carry burdens of responsibility, and by shirking those responsibilities, we are less healthy, less wealthy, and less at liberty than we could be. A moral society that fails to take charge of its health destiny only makes its health problems worse.

Currently we are hostages, trading our liberties to power structures in exchange for promises and, in the process, enslaving ourselves to them. The following chapters provide a "cure": a healthier model of health care delivery. To become a healthy society, we must radically cooperate and embrace a return to values-based medicine. This change is not merely optional; it is crucial.

References

Berwick, Donald. 2005. http://wistechnology.com/conferences/dhc

2005/Presentations/Chaiken. ppt#266, 8, Reality of Systems; cited March 31, 2007. INTERNET

Pirsig, Robert. 1991. *Lila*. New York: Bantam Books.

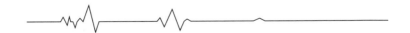

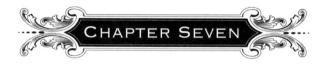

CHAPTER SEVEN

Fundamentals
of Applied Values:
Values-Based Medicine

A Basis for Agreement

PRINCIPLES

A successful health care system will expand patients'
freedom, provide services and products that are beneficial, fair, avoid harm, and preserve life. There may
be conflicts in values that will require resolution, such
as autonomy vs. beneficence, individual vs. distributive justice, and others. Any resolution of differences
should be made by putting the interests of individual
patients before the interests of the state. Collective
decisions in health care are best applied as general
guidance through principles, rather than specific
rules of conduct. The following strategy is grounded
in philosophy and has a practical and useful end: the
promotion and maximization of good through the
provision of quality health care.

UNIVERSAL ACCESS

No discussion of health care principles would be complete without acknowledgement of the necessity for
universal access to care. Whether the premise stems
from the application of principles like justice or from
the Golden Rule, all citizens should have access to

health care services. Without this common agreement, no proposal for change can begin. And as we shall see, to take any other perspective is economically wasteful. Questions about whether quality of care and principles are served if there are unequal outcomes are beyond the scope of this book.

MEDICAL OUTCOMES

A few decades ago, Scandinavian Airlines System was a state-owned and state-run enterprise that was not performing well in a competitive world. The airline was privatized. While the story may be apocryphal, Jan Carlzon, the first CEO, is said to have called the employees together and announced, "There are two and only two jobs in this company: please be sure you are taking care of a customer; and if you are not, please be sure you are taking care of someone who is." This was his "Moments of Truth" service strategy put to action.

The statement is relevant to health care, too. By substituting the word "patient" for "customer," we can agree that the first priority of health care is patient care. The resulting bureaucracy has only two levels—to care for a patient, or to take care of someone who is. This resonates with the understandings of patients, doctors, and nurses alike; in the "moments of truth"—health care encounters—the sole focus must be the patient.

The most important patient outcomes are living better and longer. Any other metrics are likely to be intermediary process outcomes or irrelevant. Individuals know when matters have become medically hopeless, so a longer life of misery is not necessarily a preferred choice. The individual can best make an informed choice about health and health care in such circumstances.

When measuring the outcome and quality of health care, having a preferred method for the evaluation and treatment of illness is important but only in direct relationship to improving the quality and/or longevity of a patient's life. Evidence-based medicine, in the aggregate, focuses on these outcomes, and values-based medicine specifically addresses these two core outcomes. Focusing on prior or intermediate outcomes, such as conformance to rules, runs the risk of stifling innovation and deflection of resources to NVAPs. There must also be an integrated concept of the economic consequences of health and health care.

Values-Based Medicine: The Essentials

The necessary components for quality health care include patient care, research, education, and prevention. Investments in professional and public education, research, and prevention are impossible to separate from quality patient care. When we invest, we should not be short-sighted about the returns on these investments.

A new option for health care will resolve the seemingly intractable problems of the current system. I call this option Values-Based Medicine (VBM). In VBM, a social contract exists between patients and caregivers. All health value-producing services should be provided to patients by caregivers; in turn, patients will be responsible for maintaining their well-being by refraining from harmful habits and behaviors. This is possible because the ultimate creators of value—both medical and economic—are human. When health care improves the life of a responsible person, he or she becomes more productive in both these senses; hence, citizens are the ultimate value production centers.

Here's how, and why, it works. Responsible patients are people who take care of themselves, proactively steer clear of hazard, and agree to participate as contributing citizens by being productive. In Part I, we explored some of the ways in which persons might not take proper care of themselves, become witting or unwitting participants in negative-value-producing behaviors (egocentric ignorance, character deficiency, and/or destructive behaviors), or simply be lazy and non-contributory. In the new option, such behaviors would not be rewarded.

The economic value of life demonstrates the opportunity to provide health services where the returns are indirect yet very real. There would be no special class of citizen for which a special program need be created or sustained. Hence, Medicare, Medicaid, VA, etc., all could potentially be part of the new, comprehensive system. The "bills," which are actually investments in projected economic returns, would be paid by a flourishing economy, which is substantially the consequence of a healthy citizenry.

Caregivers would participate by agreeing to provide services that result in two outcomes: improved quality of life and increased longevity. They would be provided a base annual salary, plus a bonus for a percentage of the economic value added (EVA) that results from their care. The concept of a team would be a necessary and firmly ingrained part of the outcome. No one physician or nurse can prosper at the expense of another since the overall welfare of the patient determines the bonuses. Base salaries, bonuses, and the method of calculation may all vary. Still, the value of life is so high that all parties to the transaction should be fairly compensated in an ongoing manner. Patients do better, the caregivers are more equitably paid, and there is a dividend—"health capital"—to society that will more than support the proposed system.

Consider the concept of health care as a family business, where we all are members of the health family. We have a long-term view of the investments to be made and a clear focus on the outcomes we desire. We know how to reward performance and to create a system to do so. The system is open for review, and each "member" receives access to finely detailed reports.

For illustration, assume that we are currently spending $2 trillion per year on health care in the United States. Let us also assume that all of that money is not being well spent, and that a substantial minimum of 60% is not being spent on value-added patient care processes. Let us further assume that of the remaining 40%, a minimal estimation of one-half of the money is spent on self-inflicted disease. In theory, that means that we are spending approximately $800 billion on patient care and $400 billion on irreducible, non-self-inflicted disease. Doctors work cooperatively with responsible patients, and all of a sudden, the "investment" requirement for the new system is cut to 20% - 40% of the current total.

We must consider the economic potential for doing a better job, as defined by meaningful outcomes. In chapter 9 we will consider in detail a "what if, doable" scenario. In this calculation, we determine the potential health dividend to the economy of improving quality of life 20% (0.05 utility point values) and increasing longevity by five years to be nearly $100 trillion in "new money" economic growth benefit. Let us assume that we will continue to spend $2 trillion per year in nominal 2006 U.S. dollars on health care, and that this will all be spent on achieving meaningful outcomes, rather than the currently wasteful and enslaving processes. In twenty years, we will have spent $40 trillion to get a return of $100 trillion. This sounds like something to consider as an investment. In fact, given the inexorable calculus of returns on investment and the savings incurred by eliminating waste, the returns are potentially much greater. If we consider David Cutler's appraisal that the economic growth potential from improvements in health for the U.S. economy approaches $1 quadrillion ($1,000 trillion or $1,000,000 billion), then health care clearly is not a cost center; it is a value production center. In short, there is and will be plenty of money to provide quality, value-added, universal health services.

If there is any concern about whether caregivers will be able to participate in this new system, here are some numbers to consider. There are about 700,000 licensed physicians in the United States. An increasingly unfortunate and dangerous trend is that not all of them care for patients, but let us assume they all did. Let us further assume that we citizens wanted to be certain that we were attracting the best, brightest, most capable, youthful minds to become doctors. We also wanted to attract these key persons to health care by rewarding them as they should be rewarded. Let us plan to pay each of them commensurately in salary and performance bonuses, where performance is measured by improvements in quality of life, longevity, and economic growth. Less than one half the amount currently being spent would provide handsomely for this critical contribution. As performance improves, the value of physicians' and nurses' services will be clear to see and compensation can rise commensurately.

The same logic applies to all other caregivers. In fact, it would be in everyone's interest that these compensations be as high as possible, again provided the investment led to improvements in the relevant patient outcomes.

Design Principles of Values-Based Health Care

In addition to the general characteristics above, Values-Based Medicine should rest firmly on very specific principles. It will have as its prime focus patients as individuals and, as such, relationships will be cooperative, not adversarial. Principles best deliver technical and moral quality; power corrupts and enslaves. Profiteering is unjust; economic consequences should be equitably applied and borne. The operational model should value dynamic quality—the creative force of innovation—with static quality "ratchet" locks to preserve the good.

The new system should minimize energy drains from our own bad behavior, over-regulation, and simple neglect. It should shift resources from positions of lower to higher value. By raising the potential energy value of our citizens and decreasing deterioration, we create a fountainhead of new resources that may be applied in a new, virtuous cycle of outcome improvements.

Finally, the model should focus on what matters most in the human context: trust. The context, or engine of value production, is human life. Dynamic quality is the spark that ignites the motor; trust sustains it. The production of the engine, and the fuel that enables it, is economic growth. Other products are cultural vitality and social tranquility. Good health—quality of life and longevity—provides an opportunity for us to be productive, happy, and free. The system should result in "medicine befitting free men," and not "slave medicine," as described by Plato.

Here, again, is the schematic for our new, simplified Values-Based Medicine health care system:

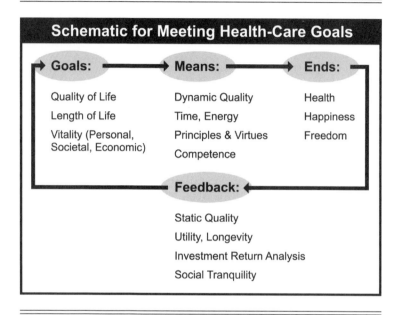

FIG. 7.1

The goals reflect the fundamental purposes of health care: (1) Help individuals live better and longer and (2) Improve the vitality of individuals and society.

The means should include enabled creative forces and resources. They begin with dynamic quality, the prime source of innovation, and proceed to basic resources of time and energy to bring the principles and virtues of competence and compassion to the endeavor.

These are the four ends to the simplified Values-Based Medicine health system:

+ Health

+ Freedom

+ Happiness

+ Goodness (in the meaning expressed by Pirsig)

Robert Pirsig summarizes his thinking about the "Metaphysics of Quality" by simply concluding: "Good is a noun." This concept has real merit in considering a values-based solution to health care. In his discussion he alludes to the use of "good" in language. If good is a noun, then it has substance beyond subjects and objects. For medicine, this would mean that "good" may be created in the relationship space between patients and caregivers. "Good" describes the valued outcome, which first enhances the patient, then affirms the caregiver, and ultimately benefits society. In other words, the substance, pattern of value or quality, called good occupies the spaces within us and between us.

The feedback loop of the Values-Based Medicine Simple System should measure that which is meaningful and provide a mechanism for preserving and improving the good created. Static quality mechanisms are put in place that improve utility and longevity, maximize the economic investment returns, and contribute to measures of a stable, tranquil society.

The system works by way of a panel of health care providers, who will agree on a new dynamic for the provision of services. They will focus on patient-centered outcomes of improved quality of life and longevity. They will take as their primary job the fulfillment of these goals. They will be rewarded with a sufficient income to sustain their practice and their lives, plus a bonus or annuity for sustained public health and economic outcomes. In effect, they will be rewarded for making patients better, not just for performing tests and procedures on patients.

The business model is like a family-owned enterprise, rather than a publicly traded company with shareholder returns as its primary objective. In this sense, long-term thinking and long-term goals can prevail. And the "returns" are enjoyed equally by everyone involved in the model. This family-owned business model ideally includes all of us and the benefits are returned to further enhance the benefits. We all will live better when we are individually healthy. Failure to invest fully in that principle limits our individual and societal potential for well-being. The dividends become self-perpetuating and the opportunities for mischief are minimized. Like all good families, we will care for one another, watch over one another, hold one another accountable, and glory in the benefits that accrue to each of our members. The outcomes will not all be equal, but the opportunities will be.

Health contracts will provide for medications and medical devices based on their demonstrated added value. There will be ample opportunities for profit in these spheres, but such profits will be tied to outcomes, as it is for doctors and nurses, rather than to marketing.

There will be major overhaul of NVAPs such as payer and regulatory processes. Dynamic quality improvements will be centered on patient care issues. Those that are not will be systematically removed from the backs of patients, doctors, nurses, and hospitals alike. In effect, care processes will be evaluated for their patient outcome performance results. One simple starting point would be to put the people with the most knowledge about the enemy (disease) and how to prevent and cure it—doctors and nurses, principally—in charge of the system and its institutions.

Options for a Values-Based Medicine Health Care System

Various options can be created to maximize a patient's autonomy of choice and provide incentives for performance outcomes that matter.

Option A-1
Full Coverage for Responsible
Adults and All Children

This option redirects the federal contribution to the pro-vision of meaningful outcomes for health care services. All value-added health services should be provided to all voluntarily participating citizens, regardless of age. No insurance policies, no non-value-added regulations, no middle persons, no non-value-added administrative paperwork—only care guaranteed by social contract between patients and caregivers, backed by a stable and independent federal bank, and funded by the current share of payroll taxes applied to health care. The core criteria are: if the service adds quality of life and longev-ity for patients, thereby increasing the economic vitality of society, and if it expands the liberties of the parties to the relationship, then that care is provided. There would be only one, non-monetary "premium" paid by the beneficiaries: they must take care of themselves and be contributing members of society.

There will be no additional "charges" for the services provided under Option A-1. Any patient under the plan will act responsibly, practice healthy habits, participate in disease prevention programs, take their medicines as prescribed, and so on.

Patients and care providers will pay for these services with their contributions to society by participating in the work force as long as they are able, paying taxes, and being good citizens. If they do not wish to participate, they will choose another option and bear its additional costs.

The indigent, those unwilling to contribute to their own care, and those who choose to purchase care independently of the option will be cared for under another model, described below in Option B.

OPTION A-2
ADDITIONAL PREMIUMS FOR BAD BEHAVIOR

Some individuals may wish to opt out of A-1 but only in part. They would like to participate to a point where their potentially dangerous or self-destructive behaviors have a calculable, additional cost, which they are willing to pay. For example, if a person chooses to become and stay morbidly obese or to smoke, he may be willing to pay the incremental cost of the burdens, or if a person refused to take her needed medicine, like those used for treating diabetes or depression, they might be willing to pay an additional premium to indulge these behaviors.

OPTION A-3
"SPA USA"

There will likely be a significant number of persons so mired in egocentric ignorance, character disorder, or destructive behavior that they will not qualify to participate in any other version of Option A. They will likely profess a litany of explanations and rationalizations and repeatedly promise they will behave, but they will not. Their sociopathy will be too controlling. We need to offer an option of redemption, a status to be earned. This redemption is unlikely to be achieved in that person's current environment, and so there should be a physical place to go for a specified time, during which the opportunity to participate in Option A is earned. This Spa USA should meet the need for various services: lifestyle management, detoxification, health education, citizenship, job training, and the like. Attending this program is optional, but participation in the program once enrolled is not. Anyone should be free to leave at any time prior to completion of the program.

OPTION B
CURRENT SYSTEM OPTIONS

Because there will likely be significant, multiple levels of resistance to change, there will need to be sufficient diversity and continuity to provide needed services to non-participants in Option A. They will, quite literally, show up on our medical doorsteps, and so options should be available, political will and resources providing. These options will be funded, as they currently are, principally at state and local levels.

OPTION B-1
COUNTY, CHARITY, OR FAITH-BASED HOSPITALS PLUS "FREE" CLINICS

These facilities are generally supported at local levels to provide services for indigent and uninsured care. There is no need to contemplate a dismantling of this system. It is likely to continue to be a necessary adjunct for those who do not qualify for any of the Options A. There is a large and profound moral legacy to these facilities and services, which is to be respected. Option A should substantially reduce the burden of these hospitals in that the responsible and productive uninsured will likely opt for A-1 services. In the economic model previously presented, doctors and nurses are already compensated, so this should substantially relieve the cost burdens of caring for the irremediably irresponsible, noncontributing residents, certain undocumented persons, or illegal immigrants.

OPTION B-2
INCARCERATION

A large component of health care services are provided under contract to those incarcerated. There are currently approximately 2.2 million persons in jails, receiving court defined and enforced care. (A total of about 7 million persons are either incarcerated, on parole, or on probation; about 2 million of the total are related to drug-related crimes.) That burden is unlikely to diminish unless we can unlock the keys to responsible behavior. There will likely be a continuing discourse about the appropriate levels of care to be afforded to these individuals; in the meantime, such care is required to be provided.

OPTION B-3
DIRECT PAYMENTS FOR SERVICES RENDERED

Some persons may be concerned that they will not receive a desired level of service, or a desired level of responsiveness from any new system. They may wish to pay out-of-pocket for services for a range of reasons, including the perceived need for immediate and personalized services, disinterest in participating in a generalized plan available to all citizens, or simply individual notions of personal liberty that include paying directly for services received. These should be available options. They are much more likely to be cost-effective in that they would be unburdened by all the current waste. It should be understood that this option is generally chosen based on the purchaser's sense of the value of the service, which often does not encompass certain pre-structural service enablers, such as education, research, and development. Accordingly, pricing for such services should appropriately reward all enabling investments, including these. Providers will be free to serve these individuals as they wish.

The Federal Health Bank

Because health care is a productive entity, creating human and economic resources, society has a compelling interest in designing a system to maximize that output. At various times, and in differing mixtures and measures, society and its representative governments are important, strategic players in health care concerns. They represent the prime, systematically interested collective parties and the best sustainable source for the investment. They are the only parties with a sufficiently long-term view of benefits and return on investment, and they are the best positioned to set the rules of engagement and verify the metrics. Finally, they are frequently the source of the solution, through wise or fortuitous action.

Accordingly, I recommend the formation of a politically independent, Federal Health Bank. The Bank will be modeled in part after the Federal Reserve Bank. The purpose would be to provide a sustainable, federal economic investment in health. Because the Bank will be an independent entity, a long-term investment model may be established and sustained. To assure operational efficiency and discipline, the Bank should enter into contracts for services (Health Service Contracts, or HSCs) that are private in the sense that political and cultural whim is buffered.

Banking Principles

The strategic goal is an optimally healthy and productive nation. The operating philosophy will be cooperative; adversarial elements will be limited to dispute resolution at local levels. The business model is comparable to a family-owned business. Citizens are free to choose how they manage their health and its maintenance, with strong incentives provided for responsible behaviors and disincentives for irresponsibility. An investment model with disciplined measurement of returns should replace the current reimbursement/cost-based system. Patient-centered added values are the prime outcomes to measure and reward. Accordingly, the objectives are value-added programs to increase quality of life and longevity and consequently maximum leveraged health investment returns through improvements in health status.

The Functions of Government

Congress, the executive branches, and federal courts will authorize the creation of the Bank and authorize the purchase of health care services through contracts (HSCs) authorized by the Bank. Government may or may not choose to continue to provide funding for health programs, including Medicare, Medicaid, or other "special class" alternatives they may wish to maintain or establish. Alternatively, Congress need no longer provide for health care services, research, or education. They may assign these roles to the new system and Bank. It may, at its discretion, transfer its authority through contracts administered by the Bank governance and consider dismantling current programs or melding Medicare and Medicaid into Option A-1, a strongly recommended option.

The Department of Health and Human Services will broadly authorize Health Service Contracts (HSCs) to provide services that add value to the health of citizens. These contracts would be horizontal to cover populations by geographic area or by common interest, or the contracts would be vertical to cover populations by specialty or disease. Contracts should require 60% operational control of operating entities by physicians and nurses providing medical care. Note that "ownership" of the assets will be irrelevant; their only purpose is to drive beneficial outcomes. Contracts may not discriminate on any basis except value-based performance or against citizens who have enrolled. All citizens may enroll in the program Option A-1, provided they behave responsibly.

Role of Providers

Providers will enter into contracts for outcomes, rather than for encounters or procedures. They can terminate or renew contracts and will be incentivized on the basis of value-added performance. Contracts will provide for health care services, health education, prevention, and research.

Role of Citizens

Individual patients may choose to participate in Option A or other alternatives of their own choice such as Options B-1 or B-3. Patients will participate by improving their quality of life and longevity through healthy living choices.

Should they decline in word or deed, they would cease to be eligible for full Option A coverage.

Role of Other Parties

GOVERNMENT AGENCIES

Current government programs in quality assurance may be suspended and the requirements rolled into contracts for services recommended at any time. Public health functions, including the Public Health Service, Agency for Research and Health Quality, Centers for Disease Control, Federal Drug Administration, certain portions of the Drug Enforcement Agency, and appropriate state programs funded by Congress, may be reconfigured to be performed under contract through the Bank and HSCs. Military health care for service branches and the Veterans Administration system may remain as presently configured, or transferred at the discretion of the services in whole or in part to the Bank and HSC contracts, to be run on a value-added basis. Non-government agencies may participate in Bank and HSC contracts and may initiate, organize, and manage aspects of those contracts, subject to limits of operational control.

THE BANK

The Federal Health Bank will initially be administered as an independent division of the Federal Reserve Bank. Congress will authorize and provide $1.1 trillion per year, approximately the current federal share of the so-called "payer-mix," plus escalators indexed to inflation per year, to fund the Bank. These funds may be obtained through a restricted offering of U.S. Government Securities for this purpose or as a direct allocation. In addition, the Bank will receive 25% of federal revenues received as a result of the incremental "health effect" growth in the economy. Since about 50% of the growth in the economy and federal revenues is the result of improvements in health, the Bank will share equally with other federal programs—25% of the health dividend to the Bank and 25% to support other programs—as dividends of success. This health dividend will be calculated on an annual basis and paid in quarterly installments to the Bank. Finally, the Bank will be capitalized with additional amounts for assuming other existing federal health programs, should their functions be transferred, such as the Centers for Disease Control, National Institutes of Health, and Federal Drug Administration, at the election of Congress and the executive branch.

States may also participate at their own election. Current health care services may be provided through the Bank and HSCs. The general model will apply here as well.

The Bank will not assume past financial liabilities or future, externally imposed liabilities. Excess funds will be used to create and grow an endowment, which will fund medical education and research, and which in turn will be rewarded with growth from the dividends they contribute to the added values of improved quality of life and longevity.

Will there be enough money to pay for all of this? Will there be dividends? Please see Chapter 8 for the answers to these and other investment questions.

Policy and Rules

Policy and rules are to be set by the Bank's governing board, which will have citizen representation. Since the philosophy is cooperative, services will be designed and contracted for the purposes of insuring success of the contracted parties in fulfilling the strategic goals. Mediation processes will exist for disputes. Legal processes, including those for termination of participation of parties and contracts, will be considered failure and are to be avoided.

References

Pirsig, Robert 1991. *Lila*. New York: Bantam Books.

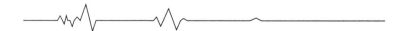

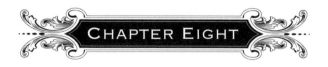

CHAPTER EIGHT

Health Care Investing

Health care qualifies for Samuel Johnson's accolade as the greatest benefit to mankind.

—William Nordhaus—

Current Investment in U.S. Health Care

The market capitalization of value of health care and health-related stocks on American exchanges is just over $2.8 trillion, representing just over one thousand listed companies. Approximately 62% of them pay no dividends and they likely have small to negative net revenue. About 51% of the total market capitalization value is made up of about 150 pharmaceutical companies, and, in all likelihood, they constitute much more of the total profit in health care.

About twenty managed care companies, 2% of the companies listed, comprise 6% of the market capitalization value. Their power and influence over the care of citizens go well beyond this relatively modest economic position. One cannot fail to reflect on the dynamic that has led so few to be able to control and limit the options of so many through such pervasive and sequestered positions of power. This system is not sustainable. The operational complications and costs of this unfathomably complex web do not favorably compare to core values of quality of life and longevity.

These numbers seem large because the positions of political and economic power and influence of these two categories are huge. Nonetheless, they pale in the face of the opportunity for value production in health and health care.

The New Investment Model

To consider health care as a cost center is severely detrimental. The potential economic dividends of improved health are so large as to stretch credulity and demand our responsive embrace.

I propose a formula for the calculation of Economic Value Added (EVA) to the US economy—new dollars added to the economy—through improvements in health status conferred by improved quality of life and increased longevity. The EVA from improvements in health and health care is on the order of $8.6 trillion per 1% improvement in quality of life and $11.1 trillion per year of increased longevity for the US population. The total EVA potential for health improvements is in the hundreds of trillions of dollars, with conservative estimates of returns on investment in the range of five to ten times.

The EVA benefits to the US economy are so large as to call into question current "cost containment" strategies for managing health care in the United States. Health care investments do not qualify as a drain on US resources; they create them. Almost any conceivable analysis suggests it is in society's best interest to find and treat any treatable disease with the most advanced methods available at the earliest possible time, at virtually any cost.

A General Perspective on
the Economics of Health Care

Consider health care as a necessary investment in a healthy economy. For the moment, leave aside the medical benefits of improved diagnosis and treatment of disease and moral notions such as right, good, beneficence, and justice. Nordhaus has calculated that approximately 50% of the growth in the US economy for the twentieth century was attributable to improvements in health and health care (Nordhaus 2006).

Still, extant economic analysis remains somewhat detached from the values system that resonates with patients, nurses, and physicians. They know that patient vitality and well-being forms the basis for the true bottom line. That line needs to be effectively connected to other "bottom lines" without shunting dollars to places that do not provide improvements in patient well-being.

A prime reference point for the US economy is the gross domestic product (GDP), a measure of the nation's production of goods and services. According to the US government, the GDP in 2005 was estimated to be $12,605.7 billion or $12.6 trillion. A number of economists, summarized by Cutler and Richardson, have calculated the economic value of an American citizen's life. The average was approximately $5 million, with the range between about $3 million and $7 million. In particular, contributions to the economy by increasing the longevity of a life were analyzed. One year of life in perfect health is worth approximately $100,000; a year of life extension is conservatively worth $75,000. The current US life expectancy at birth is 77.71 years. Note that these calculations analyze the effects of only longevity, and not of quality of life. (Cutler and Richardson 1997)

Quality of life improvements, as distinct from longevity effects, are intuitively contributory to human and economic vigor. The question whether, and to what extent, value of life calculations that are derived primarily for longevity may be integrated with quality of life effects has yet to be resolved. The approach described here proposes such a resolution. A bridging methodology is required, and the key element of that bridge is utility.

"Utility" in health care refers to the quality of life associated with a health status. Because its boundaries are zero, indicating death, and 1.0, indicating perfect health, it inherently, conceptually, and practically integrates the notions of longevity and quality of life. Utility becomes a linch pin in the calculation of economic consequence for the full range of health and health care interventions. For example, it may be calculated for an individual, group, or population; a particular health condition or all health-altering states; and as an indicator of any health intervention from public health and prevention to therapeutic methods such as pharmaceuticals and surgery. Utilities are now available for a broad range of health conditions and status, and the methods of value-based medicine are becoming standardized (Brown and Brown 2005; Center for the Evaluation of Value and Risk in Health 2001). No data exists for the mean utility of the US population, but an analysis of data extracted from the United Kingdom calculated the mean utility of that population to be 0.75. (VanPraag and Ferrer-I-Carbonell 2001). A recent report suggests that the overall health utility, or quality of American lives, may be inferior to that of England and achieved at considerably higher cost (Banks, Marmot, Oldfield and Smith 2006).

Consider the following method of computing the economic contribution of health care to the US economy. To obtain a picture of a precise way to measure the economic impact of increased longevity and quality of life on our economy, I constructed a formula of economic value that incorporates many of the known variables from research results.

Formula

A general formula for US economic value resulting from improvements in health and health care interventions is the Economic Value Added (EVA), or economic contribution:

EVA =

Value of Life (VL) x

f [improved utility (U) + increased longevity (L)]

x K1 (health effect contribution to the economy)

x K2 (proportion of life, or time of benefit effect)

– Cost (C), at time (t), for population (P),

Or, EVA = $VL \, (\triangle U + \triangle L) \cdot K_1 \cdot K_2 - C$

Where:

EVA = Additional nominal US dollars derived from improvements in health and health care.

VL = Value of life—a conservative consensus value (in 2005 US$) is $6.0 million. A snapshot value was calculated for the year 2005. Values are specified in nominal 2005 US dollars per whole population, per person (life) and per person per year (Cutler and Richardson).

U = Utility, a measure of the quality of life associated with a health status, generally derived by one of three methods: standard gamble, time trade-off, and willingness to pay.

L = The number of years that a life is extended as a consequence of improvements in health and health care.

K1 = The "health effect" coefficient, or the proportion of the growth in the economy that is attributable to improvements in health and health care. This is a theoretical factor chosen to accept the likelihood that there will not be a unit for unit economic benefit for an improvement of, say, 0.01 units of utility or per year of added life. The coefficient is likely to be multifactorial, based on the medical condition under consideration, the health status of the patient (and particularly for health states associated with very low utility), and highly non-linear. For these initial calculations, a conservative arbitrary coefficient of 0.5 was chosen.

K2 = The "life effect" coefficient, or fraction of life to which the economic effect is applied; for example, a person's quality improved at age thirty and the anticipated benefits enjoyed through the proportional remaining years of expected life, or for the years of anticipated duration of disease.

C = Cost, in nominal US dollars.

t = Time, for calculation purposes, utilizes a reference year and, therefore, is the nodal point for the "snapshot."

P = The mid-2005 estimated population of the United States is 295.7 million, and annual birth cohorts are 4.18 million live births.

Calculations are performed as if dollars and production were constant and functions are linear. Such assumptions may make the calculations more conservative looking forward. Economic growth resulting from improvements in health and health care are calculated at 50% of the total projected growth (K1). By focusing in an index year and annual effects for an average cohort, the need to discount utility gains and long-term economic gains is minimized (and consequently not calculated herein); nor is there an interest rate of return calculated or compounded for additional economic gains produced.

The results of these calculations are summarized in Figures 8.1-4. Note: the VL (GDP) is approximately 58% of the VL, indicating the method calculates the value of life to be nearly two times the GDP. Cutler and Richardson assumed value of additional years of life ($75,000 to $100,000) and, although they are variables independent of one another, correlates with the mean population utility calculated by VanPraag and Ferrer-I-Carbonelle (0.75).

VALUE OF LIFE

(IN NOMINAL 2005 US DOLLARS)

Value of Life, by Population	EVA Returns
Lifetime, whole population	$1,723.6 trillion (or $1.7 quadrillion)
Lifetime, per person	$5.8 million
Per person, per year	$75,000

FIGURE 8.1

ECONOMIC VALUE ADDED (EVA) OPPORTUNITY
IMPROVED QUALITY OF LIFE (UTILITY)
RESULTING FROM IMPROVED HEALTH

(IN NOMINAL 2005 US DOLLARS)

Utility Increments	EVA Returns
0.25 whole population @ 50% health effect (assumed utility decrement)	$215.5 trillion
0.01 whole population @ 50% health effect	$8.6 trillion
0.01 per person @ 50% health effect, per lifetime	$28,950
0.01 per person @ 50% health effect, per year	$371

FIGURE 8.2

ECONOMIC VALUE ADDED (EVA) OPPORTUNITY
INCREASED LENGTH OF LIFE (LONGEVITY)
RESULTING FROM IMPROVED HEALTH
(PER ADDITIONAL YEAR,
IN NOMINAL 2005 US DOLLARS)

One Year Longevity Effect, by Population:	EVA Returns
Whole population @ 50% health effect, per year	$11.1 trillion
Per person @ 50% health effect, per lifetime	$37,000
Per person @ 50% health effect, per year	$475

FIGURE 8.3

"What If" Scenario

If you could find a way to improve your quality of life by 20% and lengthen your life by five years, would you value that? Consider the value to you, your family, and community. Consider that you have a partnership with a caring and supporting health care system that also understands the value of your life and its contributions and is willing to invest in your future. All you must do in return is be responsible—first to yourself and then to your community. Might you be interested in that, both as an individual and as a citizen?

Consider if there were a significant breakthrough in medical understanding and/or technology or perhaps (more likely) a multi-disciplinary, comprehensive strategy to effect improvements in both utility and longevity of the American people through prevention and improved care. Imagine if that campaign's results were to create an overall improvement in population utility of 0.05 (5% overall, or 20% of the population decrement of 0.25), and increased longevity of five years. Would the reputed results warrant investment in such a program? Yes, it would! The additive effect to the US economy comes out to be about $98.5 trillion new dollars added to the economic vitality of the country. See figure 8.4.

Can you think of a better vision for the improvement in US health care than this? Let us call it five + five in twenty; five point improvement in quality of life plus five years increased longevity in twenty years. The money "earned" will surely cover the increased expenses required and leave a substantial, nearly ten times "health dividend," to the general economy to boot. Such goals are attainable.

ECONOMIC VALUE ADDED (EVA)
OPPORTUNITY OF THE "WHAT IF" SCENARIO:
INCREASED LONGEVITY OF 5 YEARS
AND IMPROVED UTILITY OF 0.05 (5%)
(IN NOMINAL 2005 US DOLLARS;
ROI = RETURN ON INVESTMENT)

"What If" Scenario Components	EVA Returns	%
Increased Longevity of 5 Years (whole population)	$55.5 trillion	58
Increased Utility of 0.05 (whole population)	$43 trillion	42
Total Scenario EVA	$98.5 trillion	ROI
(Quality of Life + Longevity)		9.9 X

FIGURE 8.4

Economic Value-Added Calculation for a Prototypical Disease: An Opportunity Calculation for Asthma

Now let us consider the following example to visualize how the model might work for a particular disease, and to calculate the total potential economic value added from the perfection of its prevention and treatment. If asthma could be eliminated from the population by a perfect technology on an annual basis, there would be significant economic benefits. Assume the following: a birth cohort of 4.18 million babies; value of life $6 million per person; a prevalence rate of 9% (372,600 of the annual cohort with the disease); a utility of 0.80 (20% quality of life decrement); an average mortality rate of 1.72 per 100,000 population; health effect (K1) on the economy 50%; a median age of onset of 30 years of age; a duration of disease of 12 years; and an annual direct cost of care of $28,000 per person per year, or $10.4 billion total cost per year in the United States. In this scenario, the potential EVA return, theoretically to be derived from the improved utility and longevity of a "perfect cure," is $133 billion, with a return on investment of 12.8 times. And these economic benefits are theoretically achievable every year, for each cohort of children born, for just this one disease! Sensitivity analysis of the formula parameters indicates the cost of care to have the smallest impact on the returns when compared to other factors, by far. Considering the leverage for EVA, there is ample justification for any and all allocations of resources that will result in improved utility and longevity in potential and actual asthma sufferers.

The example demonstrates theoretical returns, even with conservative estimates of value and generous estimations of cost. The point: health care is not a zero-sum economic exercise; it is a powerful generator of economic returns. This resonates with common sense and medical experience: to fail to do the right thing, and to prevent or reverse medical problems as comprehensively as possible, and at the earliest possible time, is bad medicine, bad social policy, and bad economics.

The Investment Case Model in a Human Context

Is it appropriate to be enthusiastic about health care spending of $2 trillion per year or 17% of GDP per year, the estimated figures for 2005? Is blaming health care for the lack of competitiveness in US manufacturing rational? An illustrative case in point is the US automobile industry. Reports regularly indicate that more money is spent on health care than steel (more than $1,500 per vehicle) and that this expenditure is the principal reason the industry cannot compete in world markets. The reality may be quite different. Humanity is an appreciating asset (negativists notwithstanding); steel is not. This fact does not suggest that all of the $2 trillion is wisely spent or that US industry must be structurally hobbled by health care expenditures in a global marketplace, whose models for health care delivery and financing differ. This analysis does propose that improved health and health care—reflected by the synergistic effects of improved quality of life and longevity—is a superb, long-term investment for people, business, and society.

Value-based calculations of the economic contributions (EVA) of health care should help to define the business case and investment strategy from all perspectives. If the default strategy is to decrease expense at all costs—which is the "cost-center" mentality for health care services—then medical outcomes become subsidiary and will surely suffer. Moreover, a business model where third-party political requirements and/or investor quarterly dividends drive the aggregate of medical decisions will inevitably compromise optimal patient care outcomes.

On the other hand, long-term investment in health outcomes, with one purpose being growth in the US economy, suggests another mindset that is driven by value. This scenario requires a continuous and consistent process of investment analysis, defining and measuring the value delivered, how it is delivered, by whom, and at what cost. Therefore, increasing the growth in the economy requires that those enterprises and people adding value to quality of life and longevity, the only meaningful desired outcomes, should be identified and enabled, while deemphasizing non-value-added structures and processes. This approach will include an independent audit of medical costs that 1) does not necessarily assume all current structures and processes add value in equal measure or even at all, and 2) informs additional investments in quality of life-enhancing and life-prolonging interventions.

The strategy of "right sizing" investments—increasing some and decreasing others—based on added values like utility and longevity—should be the appropriate result. One such "what if" scenario—improved mean population utility by 20% (0.05 utility units) and longevity by five years—appears both feasible and highly contributory to both health and wealth. Returns on investment on the order of ten times seem possible (figure 8.4) even after discounting the net present value of allocations like utility and costs across the longer terms of human life. This analysis seems to confirm an emerging sense among economists: the total value of the economic growth opportunity results from improvements in health and health care is likely to be in the hundreds of trillions of dollars.

One should question the validity of considering life and dollars as in some sense interchangeable, for example in the calculation of the GDP on a per capita basis. Is it proper to assume that there are only human contributions to the GDP and not other "engines" of production such as factories? Imagine the productivity of the "hard" assets like land, buildings, factories, and equipment if there were no people. Production would not only grind to a halt, there would be no purpose for the production; no purchasers and no consumers. The only context for any productive activity, including health care, is human. That context is relevant only for groups of humans in a society. Hence, measures of productivity apply only to human beings in a society. Therefore, the GDP is ultimately only human productivity and the calculation is reasonable.

A related question is the matter of why the estimated value of life is more than the sum of the economic activity reflected in the GDP. This relates to the nature of the GDP and what it does not include, namely the human sense of well-being. That sense includes more than the value of measured productivity and many other enrichments that add to the values humans hold dear in life:

+ Fulfilling love and friendship relationships

+ Environments of beauty

+ Liberty and equality

+ Personal and financial security

+ Intellectual pursuits like inquiry and learning

+ Good feelings like happiness and good will

+ Sensual pleasures (visual, auditory, olfactory, gustatory, tactile)

+ Spirituality

No one should be surprised that humans value their lives and these enrichments more than the sum of their raw, measured, economic productivity. That the consensus calculations of the value of life nearly doubles that of production, even in an economic analytical context, should resonate with all of us.

These calculations demonstrate the large potential for economic development to be derived from improvements in the quality of life and increased longevity. These are not new notions. What should be explored are the implications for the current system of resource applications in health care and how they should be modified. On the surface, envisioning a world in which economic sense dictates spending less on health care innovations that produce demonstrable improvements in utility and longevity seems unreasonable. For virtually any conceivable scenario, failure to make these investments appears to be a wasteful, lost opportunity and perhaps even consequentially immoral. The "what if" scenario of increasing longevity and utility by five years and 0.05 utility is a credible strategy and vision for health care for an intermediate time frame; it would likely be highly contributory to well-being, wealth, and liberty. To be sure, there are challenges that may make rational action improbable. These challenges include identifying and eliminating non-value-added processes, the political will to invest for the long term rather than spend in the short, and an investment model with a sufficiently long timeline to realize the returns. Nonetheless, it would appear that the exploration of alternative financing methods is a worthy consideration.

These calculations are likely to be conservative. First and foremost, the value-of-life calculations use reference analyses that ascribe growth in the US economy to increased longevity alone. In fact, there are almost certainly substantial additional contributions that result from increased quality of life, hence the use of the additive equation here. This may understate the total value of life—and the economic opportunity—by a factor of 30% to 42%. Second, the value-of-life numbers are calculated using economic reference data from the early-to-mid-1990s; the economy has grown substantially since that time. Hence the method might assume a higher dollar value of life per year in 2005 than in 1997. In short, the EVA is calculated based on assumptions that may substantially understate the potential for economic growth that results from improvements in quality of life and longevity.

The concepts and assumptions underlying the proposed formula should be tested against additional data and perspectives. This tool, and the analyses that go with it, are intended to spur that discussion. The potential uses of the derivative calculations are multiple. It may be inherently interesting to know the degree to which health and health care contribute to the economy, and the results may be useful to guide business and social policy. Such knowledge may guide health investment decisions by determining what and who adds value to health outcomes and to what extent. The tool may be useful in guiding investment resource allocations and in aligning incentives with desired outcomes where it is clear that desired medical outcomes lead to significant economic returns. On the other hand, even if and when it can be unequivocally determined that relatively small invest-ments pay large dividends, there can be no guarantee that this understanding will lead to wise decisions.

The contribution (EVA) to the US economy that results from improvements in health and health care is very large, and the potential for economic return is huge—on the order of five to ten times and scores of trillions of dollars within intermediate time frames. Using two methods of calculation—the effects on the GDP and the more inclusive assessment of the value of years of perfect health—the benefits are so large as to call into question our current strategies for managing health care in the United States. Health care investments do not qualify as a drain on US resources; they (investments in health) cause them (resources, "goods") to proliferate. Patients and providers alike should strongly consider this new strategy for care and call for replacement of the current model with the recommended health care system.

References

Banks, James, Michael Marmot, Zoe Oldfield, and James P. Smith. 2006. "Disease and Disadvantage in the United States and in England." *JAMA* 295:2037–45.

Brown, M.M, G.C. Brown and S. Sharma, 2005. *Evidence-Based to Value-Based Medicine.* Chicago: AMA Press.

Center for the Evaluation of Value and Risk in Health. Preference Weights, 1988-2001. http://www.tufts:nemc.org/cearegistry/data/default.asp. Cited March 20, 2007. INTERNET

Cutler, D. and E. Richardson. 1997. "Measuring the Health of the US Population." Brookings Papers on Economic Activity: Microeconomics. <http//www.laskerfoundation.org/reports>

Nordhaus W.D. 2006. "The Health of Nations: The Contribution of Improved Health to Living Standards." 17 Nov. 1999. <http//www.laskerfoundation.org/reports>

Stammler, Jeremiah. M.D.
Stammler worked at the Chicago Board of Health in the 1960s. I had the privilege of being a summer intern

at the Board and to be exposed to his voice of reason and wisdom. He was one of the earliest to determine that on average, the life expectancy for pack-a-day smokers is about 9 years less than non-smokers. Smokers might rationalize that losing 9 years off the end of their life, when they are elderly, is negligible, but Stammler understood that in fact those 9 years physiologically affect and diminish the middle years of their lifespan, and not the end years. Hence the derivative logic is valid that extending life is valuable for health care and particularly the younger (sooner) the better. Since the value is primarily captured in the robust middle of productive life, the economic consequences are not negative in relationship to current social entitlement programs.

Van Praag, BMS, and A. Ferrer-I-Carbonell. 2001. "Age-differentiated QALY Losses." Tinbergen Institute Discussion Paper (TI 2002-015/3). http://www.tinbergen.nl

<http//:www.bea.gov/bea/dn/gdplev.xls>
INTERNET

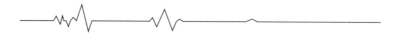

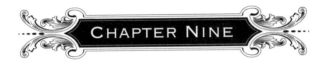

CHAPTER NINE

Building a Coalition and Overcoming Resistance

No solution to the health care crisis can work without the active engagement of those with the most vested interests in being healthy: we, the people. We must recognize both our contributions to our problems and their solutions. Anything else is a waste of energy, resources, human potential, and economic opportunity. The negative drains on our resources include egocentric ignorance, character disorders, and destructive behaviors, all of which may cause health problems that are preventable. We must not inflict this burden of disease on ourselves. We can cut the burdens of treating disease in half by simply behaving well.

Who Should Be for It

The coalition of persons and groups who should be interested in this new approach to health care should be broad and include:

+ Citizens who value quality of life and longevity

+ Taxpayers

+ Families

+ Employers and business owners

+ Politicians

+ Health care professionals

Who Will Likely Resist

Resistors are likely to be those with a strong, vested interest in the power and money they receive from health care dollars and the current methods of acquiring more of them. They include:

+ Certain executives and shareholders in medical-related enterprises

+ Persons who do not care for patients or assist those who do, yet receive rewards for controlling them

+ Corporate medical enterprises

+ Some bureaucrats

How to Overcome Resistance

Resistance is inevitable. It will likely flow from perceived threats to some current "stakeholders" whose value additions are negative or negligible in a values-based system. Every discussion about health care reform has had to attend to an essentially political and self-interested analysis of what change will mean to them. Are these interests legitimate? The answers lie in underlying assumptions about entitlement to career, rewards, and perceptions of self-worth.

A potential example would be an insurance company. What if this proposed solution substantially replaced the need for so-called health insurance? We have explored the very limited sense in which these contracts actually relate to health. In reality, the system functions as a highly profitable cash transfer system from nominal beneficiaries to insurance company employees, executives, and shareholders. There is precious little evidence that health is improved in meaningful ways by the presence of an insurance policy, as opposed to the presence of a nurse, doctor, hospital, or applied health technology.

One might respond to insurance industry resistance by first asking them to justify their wealth transfer system on moral grounds. Then they should demonstrate in precise detail how their presence in the venture adds quality and length to your life that could not be achieved more effectively with a simplified system. Finally, they should justify the annual incomes that insurance company executives count in multiples of seven and eight figures, while your nurses and doctors count annual incomes in five figures and low six figures. As patients, we need to feel that these numbers are equitable and that these numbers serve our ultimate self interests. Unfortunately, insurance companies excel in just that kind of rhetorical and political engagement and they have the resources and vested interest to sustain it . . . ferociously.

The ultimate test is whether health care is to be viewed as an entitled jobs-and-profit preservation plan, with the political bartering that serves it, or a best use of available resources to improve patient care. As to the issue of jobs, there will be plenty of need for good people to care for patients in all kinds of ways that elevate the lives of their fellow citizens, rather than tax them. As to the middle issue of profits for insurance company executives and shareholders, if they can sell their products profitably, so be it. Senior executives and shareholders will not easily permit the wealth they are currently receiving to be threatened by alternatives. Nonetheless, we should not accept that we must inevitably accept a conspiring group of insurance companies, shepherding bureaucrats, restrictive regulations that bar entry, and cozy political alliances that infringe on our liberty. If and when change appears to be possible, we should look past the bombast to consider the merits of the ideas, rather than the noise made by the arguing.

The pharmaceutical industry's contribution to the health of Americans and the world is unquestioned. Their economic power is astounding. Their ability to navigate in a highly charged political environment is amazing. Their ability to acquire sequestered status is astonishing. There are, however, flaws in the system, and they know it. A surprisingly huge amount of money is spent on marketing; far more than on research and development. The pipeline for innovative ideas is thin, and as a consequence, there are too many minor variations on existing drugs being developed.

Whether any value analysis beyond high shareholder returns and executive compensation takes place is open to debate. There are real concerns about whether the pharmaceutical industry can continue on its present course spending so heavily on marketing, and spending relatively spotty amounts on patient care results. Who will be the first to change? This complex industry adapted so well to its economic model, and it was equally successful in its ability to navigate the halls of power and money influence. How would it navigate in an environment that more directly rewards the value-based outcomes for individual patients and society when those outcomes are measured in terms other than dollars? To be sure, there will be rewards in dollars to be earned, probably even more than now, but getting from here to there is an open question. There is a chance that this industry will be open to doing better by creating greater good along a different path. If they are not open to such change, then their opposition to values-based medicine will be formidable.

Government and its agencies are very conservative in the sense that there is tight adherence to a rigid canon of beliefs with little room to move. Their formula is the adversarial model on steroids. A proposal such as this new one will need to navigate a sea that is mined with entrenched interests. In all of the branches—Congress, executive, judicial, bureaucracy, and enforcement arms—there are multiple islands of perceived "ownership" of health care. In some cases, there are both egos and job security at issue. It is the epicenter of a medical-industrial-political complex, rife with codependency among public and private interests, including private monetary support for campaigns and their preservation of authority. These relationships are not necessarily matters of record, but the alliances are well-oiled and function with smooth, informal understandings.

On the other hand, there is no question that there are problems. And government abhors problems that result from inflexible, narrow-minded proponents, and particularly the embarrassment that follows them; such matters are political poison.

Let us focus on the ways in which this solution solves apparently intractable political problems, such as the sustainability of Medicare and Medicaid. Many of these problems boil down to money, so solutions must evolve that stabilize the fiscal challenge and do so in a way that creates political capital, thereby buffering the political branches from the embarrassment of failure. The general appeal of values-based medicine promises to be broad. Recent efforts to pass off responsibility to private, market-based strategies have struggled at multiple levels: the cash drains have intensified, the system is not working, and the political environment of health care is deteriorating.

All of this seems to be funneling toward a single-payer, government-sponsored system. As much of the world has experienced, this will most likely lead to a system that limits choice, constricts innovation, and inevitably leads to rationing. This proposal is designed to avoid these probabilities. Still, there will be challenges to egos and political canons of belief. In contrast, most of the people involved have a strong sense of public service, or they would not be where they are. There will be plenty to do that is truly beneficial and all willing hands will be needed.

Layers of bureaucracy have accumulated within the provider system. Whether they exist to fend off raids by payers, regulatory requirements, and legal threats, or whether they exist simply to manage to keep the doors open, they do exist. Accordingly, there is a large cadre of professional managers of providers, including hospitals, whose jobs may be called into question if there are only two jobs—taking care of patients or taking care of someone who is. How these persons will respond will be of interest. More likely than not, their current world view is somewhat conflicted. On the one hand, they may view caregivers as persons who serve, but on the other hand, providers may be viewed as labor requiring management. In any case, there will be more egos to preserve, and sometimes princely compensation packages to safeguard. These tensions are longstanding. I have the optimistic sense that the provider communities share a fundamental commitment to patient welfare. They may differ as to perspectives, but the discussions should be civil. In the event of substantial changes—simplification of processes, paring excessive regulation and NVAPs—there should be enhanced career satisfaction. Of one thing we can be certain: change is coming, one way or another.

A Workable Health Care System

To create a health care system that meets our expectations, we must get back to some rather simple concepts and stick to them. These solutions fall into three categories:

1. A workable system that serves the best interests of individual patients.

2. An economic model that fosters and rewards healthy people.

3. A cultural and political milieu that supports these changes.

Such a system is comprised of a simple paradigm of goals, means, ends, and feedback that features the only two meaningful medical outcomes—quality of life and longevity—that matter, while focusing on the only two jobs that add value in health care—taking care of patients and taking care of those who do.

The underlying premise of this "simple system" is that values must be the driver, and power structures, if and when they are needed at all, must be placed in service to those values. Power and money, viewed and sought as ends, are corrupting and enslaving. When we permit and reward intermediary, low-value-added and non-value-added "stakeholders"—other than the patient and the caregiver—to the medical relationship, we create wasteful anomalies. Placing power in service to values avoids parasitic and predatory waste centers.

Two Outcomes

In the flurry of discussions about evidence-based medicine, values-based medicine, pay-for-performance, disability scales, and a library full of acronyms for quality promotion, assurance, and measurement, a simple fact is obscured—the purpose of health care is to make patients feel better for as long as possible. Living better and prolonging meaningful human life have extremely beneficial effects in both human and economic well-being. Healthy people are happier, more productive, wealthier, and freer than those who are ill.

Two Jobs

In health care, there are only two jobs that will result in the meaningful outcomes. So if you are in health care, please be sure that you are taking care of a patient. If you are not, please be sure you are taking care of someone who is taking care of a patient. If you are a patient, please ask these questions of those who surround you: Are you caring for me? Are you caring for someone who is caring for me? If not, why are you here?

A Principled Economic Model

Supporting the type of health care system we are describing with adequate funding will require a robust effort. It will require energy, especially that highly concentrated form called money. It will require that health care operate as a value production center, not a cost center, and it will use a family business as an investment model in its structure, as opposed to a publicly traded company.

Energy Flux

There are only three universal components of the universe: energy, matter, and time. They are interdependent. As best we know, energy and matter are practically infinite. In health care, time is a relatively fixed commodity, and a critical determinant of the delivery or right timing of interventions of services and the outcomes, which are quality-through-time based. The energy and matter issues are more complex. We humans are production and storage units for energies of all sorts: intellectual, physical, and emotional. All of them may be used for good or bad.

Each of us has individual responsibilities to harbor these energy resources and not waste them. It must start with the individual. The sum of the parts can only be maximized by the optimization of individual citizens. Money has no meaning other than that given to it by humans in the context of a society, and money has no meaning beyond the years we choose to give it. Its value approaches zero if we are dying, and generally, we would trade all we have of it to be well.

Value Production Centers

The dominance of cost in the discussion of health care, and the anomalies this perception creates in economies, societies, and human behavior is pervasive. This is a classic example of a false premise creating amazing waste, in terms of both current practice and lost opportunity. It is wrong by 180 degrees. This perspective creates tremendous disadvantages based on ability to pay, which in turn foster the development of power enforcement and money-making schemes that diminish the autonomy of the key participants—patients and caregivers. The inevitable and progressive institutionalization of these thought processes makes them formidable barriers to solutions. We now know that health produces wealth rather than consuming it. We have the opportunity to create a new values-based system, a "re-value-ation" of health care.

Cooperate for Meaningful Outcomes

Medical care works best as a cooperative venture. Competition as a paradigm for the delivery of health care is a notion with fundamental flaws:

1. It marginalizes and subjugates the central figures—patients and caregivers.

2. It invites short-term thinking and investment.

3. It generally results in zero-sum thinking and strategy.

4. It wastes resources in fighting battles, rather than achieving results.

5. It creates victims, dependent on others.

Money should not be permitted to be an end in health care. As highly concentrated energy, money is a means to meaningful outcomes. Cooperation among the parties that actually add value to the relationship avoids these flaws.

Much of the discussion about possible health care solutions includes stimuli for market-based competition. It will not work because the price is too high and the underlying philosophy is incompatible with the endeavor. Competition requires a framework of rules and enforcement to limit the degree of "illegal" behaviors. Profits go to parties indirectly involved. The burdens quickly overcome the benefits. Rules are applied and require the acquiescence of everyone, including patients and their caregivers. The rules become compliance burdens. Rules are designed to constrain the business practices of intermediaries, to assure that they do not take too much advantage, but this rarely works to the benefit of patient care. In sum, this "managed" competition, which is excessively regulated, is too costly and too wasteful. Any system so designed for adversarial relationships is simply something to be avoided in health care, which is, by nature, a cooperative art. Patient care is diminished by this juggling act among masked adversaries of core values.

Invest in the Family Business

To align incentives with desired outcomes, and to avoid wasting resources and opportunities on non-value-added processes, a new investment model is required. The best business model is neither a government-sponsored entitlement nor a for-profit, investor-owned corporation. One makes all subservient to a political system, whose stock in trade is political power and its sustenance. The other is driven by short-term profit and shareholder returns. Both are enslaving. A family business model, broadly constructed, sees all citizens as part of the health care family. Some provide services, others require them, and each is responsible for maximizing their contributions. The family is constructed of individuals and is not some shadowy structure created to respond to goals tangentially related to health. The view is long-term, and the benefits accrue to each and all. Since the benefits are substantial, particularly if each bears responsibility for their own behaviors, the system is not only sustainable, it is contributory. In short, the business is very profitable, for good.

Conclusion: Getting Health Care Right

There are three things we must first get right for our culture to support a sustainable health care system:

1. We must be responsible for our own actions and contributions to our "family."

2. We must make health care a cooperative, not an adversarial, enterprise.

3. We must be in charge of the choices of whether and how we will have access to "medicine befitting free men," instead of our current trend of being "slaves to medicine."

Plato presaged much of what we are doing to ourselves today. We are focusing on the wrong results. Foundationally, there should be limited need for a cash-based reimbursement system for processes, procedures, or other interventions, if rewards follow meaningful outcomes. Healthy persons become more productive. When they do, the returns to society in economic vigor will pay many times over for all needed and useful services. The system will pay for itself and will be supported by economic growth. In return, only one thing is required—the responsible behavior of each of us.

Choose medicine befitting free men. The solution provided is moral, effective, and efficient. That is the reason we should start with a coalition of the willing. There will be no shortage of physicians enthusiastic to rejoin the ethical practice to which they were attracted and for which they were trained. They, and those of you who are their patients, will not miss the hassle of rules and regulations. Go when needed to the doctor, take your medicine, and behave; no "charges" will apply. The productive outcomes will fuel the resource needs of the system.

Will there be resistance? Of course, because those power structures that profit from control over others, or are rewarded handsomely for it, will not go quietly. In turn, we must demonstrate our commitment to patient care and its beneficial outcomes.

Will they win? Can they keep us from serving your interests? Not in the long run. Good will prevail sooner or later; sooner would be better.

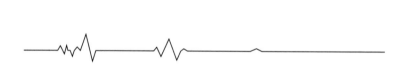

Index

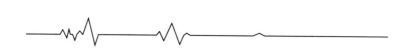